Texas Doc

More Critter Stories in the Life of a Town 'n Country Vet

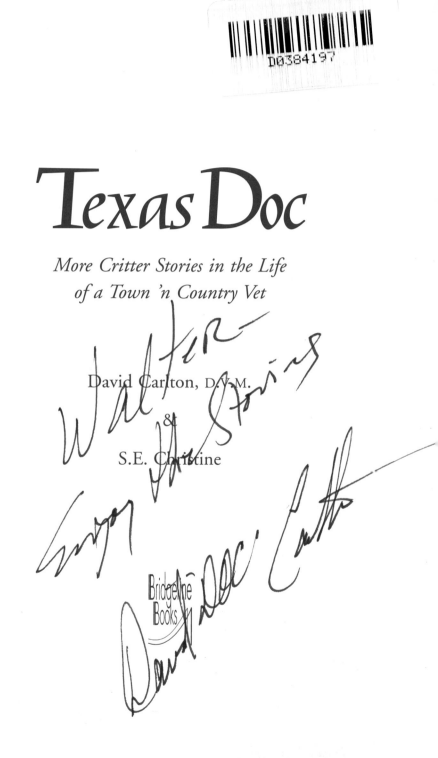

David Carlton, D.V.M.

&

S.E. Christine

Bridgeline Books

FIRST EDITION

Designed and produced by Graffolio, La Crosse, Wisconsin.
Printed by Hignell Book Printing, Ltd., Winnipeg, Manitoba, Canada.

Cover artwork from an original pencil drawing entitled 'Pals'.
Copyright © by Sheri Greves-Neilson. Information and other works
can be seen on the artist's website: grevesneilson.com

Library of Congress Cataloging-in-Publication Data

Carlton, David, 1949-
    Texas Doc: more critter stories in the life of a town 'n
country vet / David Carlton – 1st ed.
        p. cm.
    ISBN 1-888843-01-2 (pbk.)
        1. Carlton, David, 1949- 2. Veterinarians–Texas–Dallas–
Biography. 3. Veterinary medicine–Texas–Dallas–Anecdotes.
I. Title.

SF613.C37 A3 2003
636.089'092—dc21
[B]

                                                    2003048179

To my wife, Karen, and son, Kyle

And to our clients, four-legged friends,

and veterinarians…everywhere

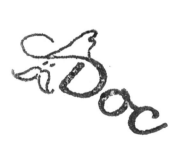

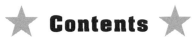# Contents

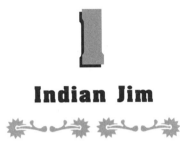

Indian Jim

bout to give up on waiting for someone to pick up the phone at Seven Star Ranch…I finally heard an unmistakable, hoarse voice answer, "Yea?"

"Uncle Grump…I'm callin' to see how Aunt Sadie's doin' 'cause you said she's having dizzy spells."

"No dizzier than normal," he replied. "And, sonny, I hear' dya be goin' out to my friend John's place to examine his new terrier…"

"Nope…his wife Maria is bringing the puppy here to Dallas instead."

A lot like brothers, John and my uncle were cut from the same mold…and had been friends forever. Similar in character and attitude, they also shared an exasperating trait: neither listened to what anyone else had to say. On top of that, no matter how many years had gone by, they both treated me like I was still a kid.

Each had been raised along Blackwater Draw at the Salt Fork of the Brazos River, where my uncle remained to become a cattleman with a small band of working cow ponies. Taking a different direction, John moved out of the county to attend college, then spent years as an accountant for a large electronics corporation in Houston. Retiring early and settling in San Angelo, he decided on a dramatic life-change—and began raising sheep.

John, dark-skinned, tall and muscular, was half Comanche. And although his proper name was Jonathan James Nogala, most folks called him 'Indian Jim'—a nickname he'd had since grade school. If his birth mother had also given him an Indian name...he kept it to himself. Proud of his heritage, he continued to keep his hair quite long and loosely tied at the back of his neck in the traditional manner. His unusually deep-set brown eyes gave John an ancient look.

Running out of anything else to say, my Uncle Grump took up his favorite topic...the weather. "Hav'ya seen the mornin' sky? Maria calls it a 'Squaw's Heaven.'" I didn't know what he was talking about, although both the sun and moon were surrounded by a blue haze.

"Storms, sonny...storms," he said. "You best be gettin' to John and Maria's before it starts rainin' pitchforks and armadillo eggs...and you can betcha the hail'll be the size of my fist."

As usual, my uncle hadn't been listening when I told him Maria was coming to Dallas. But I understood him. His mind was only on the weather. When John called, that's what he was thinking, too. "We're fixin' to have a rock-throwin', frog-stranglin', gully-washer." Neither man bothered with good grammar—but both were speaking the same West Texas slang.

Similar storms were brewing more than twenty years ago, when I had my introduction to John and the Mud River range. I couldn't help but reflect on all the confusion that resulted during that first encounter…simply because I'd never heard of the 'Indian Jim' reference. All I knew was that John and Maria were my uncle's good friends. I'd been wanting to meet Maria, since Aunt Sadie always spoke fondly of her, saying she was a gentle, 'proper' lady—a small, blue-eyed brunette from Lubbock, whom John met in college. In fact, Maria was the one to call me during the '80s requesting my help. Two hundred of their lambs on the prairie had been beaten to death by large, icy pellets of hail. "But, Doc," she added, "…that's not the worst of it…we've lost nine hundred ewes and six rams in the last few weeks to some kind of disease. Can you come out here?"

Caught up in the memories, I found myself telling Uncle Grump the story of that initial and unforgettable visit to his friend's ranch. It's a story I've told him a dozen times before—if only to needle him again for all the embarrassment I felt at not being told Indian Jim and John were one and the same person. "While driving around those dense, mesquite thickets and over the desolate, rock-infested mesa…there was no telling just how big the Mud River Ranch actually was. Fence lines were miles apart, and the rough, barren land appeared to be open range." Though my uncle grumbled as I reminisced, I rambled on:

"Dust had been blowing from the sky like sheets of rain, and my throat was drier than cotton. I finally spotted three men on horseback, and assumed they were ranch hands. They looked to be Mexican, although one may have been an Indian. Accompanied by three Border collies, they were following a flock of Angora goats and hundreds of black and white Suffolk ewes, heading toward cedar-post pens at the mouth of a long draw.

Getting closer, I noticed one of the Mexicans had a pretty fancy saddle trimmed with silver conchos. The other was riding bareback on a short, shaggy burro. Stopping Ol' Blue, and waving to get their attention...I saw that the Indian had jumped off his mustang mare to close one of the corral gates.

'Where's Maria?' I yelled, expecting one of the *caballeros* to answer. Instead, the Indian swung into his old, cavalry-leather saddle and, without a word, pointed toward a house on the far horizon.

'Who heads this outfit?' I hollered again. The Indian pointed to his chest, and rode closer. Unsmiling and appearing to be mid-age, he was wearing a crumpled straw hat shoved down over his long black hair. A makeshift rope belt hung at his waist. At the sight of his torn shirtsleeve, I thought the poor fellow probably had no money or clothes to call his own. And I wondered why Maria and John couldn't pay him more.

'*You're* the foreman?' I asked. '...and your name is?' Sliding from his saddle, he motioned for the two other hands to round up a small herd of mares gathering on the edge of the arroyo. Then he ambled over to me.

'They call me Indian Jim.' His voice was so low, I could barely hear him. He sure didn't seem like much of a foreman to me, and he didn't answer my first question...so I wasn't impressed. At this point, I still had no clue the man was Maria's husband. When I nodded, he said, 'The *señora* is preparing our chuck.'

Assuming he was referring to a chuck-wagon lunch, I knew there'd be *carne seco* or jerked beef, tepid coffee, cold biscuits. beans and 'lick'—sorghum molasses. The somber-faced man asked, 'You will join us?'

I agreed to meet him for lunch…and assumed I'd be joining him and the other hands at the bunkhouse after my appointment with John and Maria.

Raising both hands toward his lead dog, he called, 'Lobo, take Doc to *la casa*. We'll look at the sheep after *ceña. Adios*.' I soon found out that Lobo, this remarkable herding dog, had an uncanny way of understanding not only English, but every Spanish word spoken to him.

Lobo ran in front of Ol' Blue until I got close enough to see how massive the hacienda actually was. The collie, accustomed to being in control, then took off toward the stables by himself…presumably to nap after his morning of work.

Stunned to see such a magnificent home in the middle of that bleak country, I was in awe at what had been built from nothing. Technology—and money—had provided irrigation to surrounding acres now able to sustain vast fruit orchards. Stone trails wound through gardens of verbena and geraniums. And iron trellis-archways decorated the expansive wraparound porches of the Spanish hacienda with its classic red-tiled roof. A large, unusual knocker on the entrance door was actually a matador's spur. After using it, I assumed the dull, clunking sound would echo throughout the inside corridors. When there was no answer, I started to use my fist instead. But at that moment, the oak door opened. A lovely, petite woman—looking dressed for a formal occasion in a tan linen suit—greeted me.

With pronounced sophistication, the lady said, 'Please, *señor,* do step inside. I'm delighted to see you…and thank you for coming. I'm Maria.'

Put off by her regal manner, I didn't know whether to shake her hand formally or not. So I did what came naturally …tipped my brim and took hat in hand.

Inside the parlor, my eyes tried to take in everything at once. The domed ceiling of blue stained glass must have been sixty feet high. Murals depicting historical events in Texas lined the walls. And an inlaid mosaic floor-map of the state provided the entrance to what appeared to be a well-appointed, stately library. Extending the full length of the lower floor was an atrium full of noisy parrots and multi-colored, exotic birds and plants. Across from the atrium, double doors to an enormous dining room stood open. Glancing inside, I realized this was going to be a right smart affair. The lengthy mahogany table could have seated forty…and it was already set with splendors suitable for a president's banquet. I later learned it had been preset for a business dinner John would be hosting that evening.

The ranch hand calling himself Indian Jim arrived at the front door, apologizing for being late. This confused me and I wondered why he'd come to the main house. But Maria said, 'You're here. Splendid…come and join us.' She must have been expecting him.

As I awkwardly stood in the hallway waiting for Maria's husband, John, to arrive, she motioned for both Indian Jim and me to follow her into the dining room and take our chairs.

Figuring the owner of the ranch would be late, I happily settled down to enjoy the sumptuous feast of garnished roast beef, potato dumplings, mushroom risotto, and baby asparagus. There were more forks, plates and crystal glasses than I knew what to do with—but I managed.

When the Indian tied his linen napkin around his neck, I looked over at Maria, thinking she'd disapprove of his manners. But her gentle smile didn't change, and I began to wonder how often she invited this fellow to lunch.

Quietly, Indian Jim said, 'Doc...I'll show ya the worst flock as soon as we finish eating.'

'How many have ya lost?' I asked.

Maria intervened, 'Gentlemen, there will be no talking about ranch business during our meal. I'll pour your wine now.'

Ignoring her, the Indian went on to answer me. 'We've lost 'bout a thousand...I'd guess, Doc. So we still have 'bout twenty-nine thousand.'

I about choked, thinking I might be right...maybe he really was the foreman of this thirty-thousand-head sheep operation.

When Maria scolded him again, the Indian considerately obliged. 'Yes ma'am...I'm sorry.' Then, taking a few gulps of the fine '87 cabernet, and pushing his chair back...he stood up to untie the napkin and wipe his mouth. Nodding toward Maria and mumbling, 'Thank you for the fine meal,' he lumbered out of the room, saying, 'Doc, come with me.' I would have preferred to linger over wine and dessert, but I obediently followed the tall fellow outside.

Looking out over the ranch, pointing toward the south, Indian Jim said, 'Doc, my herd is down yonder. But the graveyard's way down on the west side.'

'Let's look at the living first,' I said, stressing my need to prioritize.

He referred to the herd as 'my' herd, which was strange. This would have been the right time for me to ask for clarification, since I was becoming uncomfortable. After all, I'd come here specifically to make arrangements with John, the accountant, whom I thought would be paying for my services. I was sure this poorly dressed Indian didn't have a penny.

Lobo and I tagged along as Indian Jim proceeded on foot to the sickly flock of sheep. There were several herds, but the three thousand ewes and lambs of this small herd were crowded in a canyon slue—and half of them were ill. Many were showing similar clinical symptoms. Their jaundiced mucous membranes and dull, yellow eyes caught my attention first. Other consistent signs, though not diagnostic, were depression, swollen stomachs, 'bottle jaw' edema, and anemia.

Direct and to the point, Indian Jim simply asked, 'Well, Doc...why are they dying?'

I didn't have an answer. There were more sheep here than I'd ever seen in one place. Extensive therapy, as well as laboratory and autopsy fees, would result in insurmountable costs.

'Lemme see the graveyard,' I said.

After hiking back to the ranch, we jumped into the Indian's beat-up Jeep with its missing fender and drove at least ten miles over rugged terrain to the out-of-the-way area. And I found out why it was so remote. Stopping on the rim of a small hill, the Indian didn't have to show me the carcasses in the gully below—the horrible stench did that. But I made my way down to the terrible site and viewed what looked like the tragic aftermath of some type of war. A long, narrow pit was full of decomposing bodies. Some were covered with lye, a few were half-buried, and the more recent dead were stacked at one end of the mass grave.

Needing to work on the most recent to die, I dragged two ewes and a lamb, as well as a goat and a ram, from the ditch. My stomach was churning as I took my autopsy knife in hand to begin. If I hadn't thought to include a facemask in my medicine bag, it's not likely I could have gotten through the procedures. Not knowing if gender, breed, or age were factors, I decided to do an internal inspection of random dead.

After opening and examining one belly at a time, I began to suspect the problems were liver-related. My tentative diagnosis was Black Disease or infectious hepatitis, caused by a soil-borne bacteria. I was surprised, though, to find such large numbers of wandering liver flukes in bleeding wounds.

Having remained at the top of the rise, Indian Jim hollered, 'Hey, Doc, whad'ya find?'

'God, Jim…this is weird. I've never seen liver flukes in this type of dry, desert environment. It's a serious situation. This type of parasitic migration and tissue damage can lead to deaths in epidemic proportions.'

Climbing up to the spot where Indian Jim was waiting, I showed him my knife blade with a mature, leech-resembling creature on it.

'See? Frankly, I'm dumbfounded. How did these sheep get swampy liver flukes? How?'

While I was mystified, the Indian wasn't. With a groan, he lowered his head. 'I jus' bought six thousand head from the Mississippi Delta.'

That was it...the answer. Now we needed a solution. Thousands of animals had to be saved from the disease. I racked my brain to remember the life cycle and treatment for liver flukes. While penicillin, quarantine, and vaccines would limit the bacterial devastation, the flukes still had to be eliminated.

The eggs of the fluke are passed through sheep feces to infect snails, where they multiply until they eventually emerge onto aquatic vegetation. When an animal eats the leaves, the ingested flukes mature to migrate through the intestinal walls, penetrating and destroying the liver. The bacteria then act as secondary invaders to finally become the main cause of death.

To this day, I know of no other ranch where so many thousands of sheep are raised. Small flocks were scattered over the vast, arid prairie. Fortunately, Indian Jim never mixed the new herds from the Delta with his old herds. But while most of the sheep were safe from exposure, each animal still had to be vaccinated. Around every bend and down every arroyo, there'd be another flock penned in corrals. With such vast numbers to manage, the ranch employed three shepherds to live on the range year-round. It was necessary for them to move from one grazing area to another, so their small, 'nomad' homes resembled the types of covered shepherds' wagons used throughout the world for centuries. I've seen some American ranches, though, using mobile homes or RVs for the same purpose.

I needed to quickly recruit some part-time staff to help with these mass inoculations. Indian Jim and the other two hard-working hands, Paco and Tujuillo, would also be helping.

Every morning, I brought in a new shipment of medical supplies. And whenever they could get away, either Tracy or Dr.

Vest came in with me to assist. We began vaccinating everything with four legs. We'd orally drench the fluke-infested sheep with Oxyclozanide and then treat those already having the disease with penicillin and supportive fluid therapy.

Our daily work took on an automatic, rapid rhythm of its own…and I came close to vaccinating Paco and myself twice. All of us began seeing black and white dots in our sleep. But painstakingly, one-by-one, each animal was being treated. When a tiny, twelve-week-old, orphaned lamb died as I held her, it served to strengthen my will to keep on going. But day after day rolled by before there were any noticeable effects from all our efforts. I couldn't be sure if we were winning the war or not.

During the fourteen-day battle, there were three hundred casualties. We worked as fast as we could, but the disease seemed relentless. Since Indian Jim showed up every day in the same old clothes, I was convinced we were on a shoestring budget. It also didn't help when he announced no money would be paid until our mission was complete. However, one thing impressed me about the man. Unlike many ranchers I'd known, Indian Jim appeared to personally mourn each animal's death…grieving as though a thousand more would die in the epidemic.

The fifteenth day was a good one—there were no deaths. Over twenty-eight thousand sheep were alive and recovering, although a few goats had escaped the roundup. Worn and exhausted—as we all were—the Indian just mumbled, 'We'll catch 'em later, Doc. Please bring your bill up to the house this afternoon.'

The siege had been costly—physically, mentally, and financially. And I didn't know what or whom to expect when I again used the spur doorknocker to announce myself at Maria's home.

The door was ajar, and Indian Jim called out, '*Buenos dias, Doctore* …come in, we're in the library.' Lobo ran to meet me and, gently pulling on my pant-leg, walked alongside as I sauntered in under the flags and across the mosaic map of Texas on the foyer floor. I halted for a moment at the library, astonished at the scene before me. Nothing here fit my expectations.

Wearing a silky-green lounge outfit, Maria sat curled up on the soft, leather armchair sipping from a sherry glass, while Indian Jim slowly walked back and forth behind a hand-carved, antique desk. From a small, clothbound book, he was reading poetry to Maria.

I stood frozen in the doorway, not knowing what to do. Then, clearing my throat, I boldly walked up to the desk, handing Jim my three-page invoice. At the same time, I tried to glance at the name of the poet on the tiny edition held in his hands. I couldn't make it out, but I did notice three or four checkbooks scattered over the top of the desk…and cynically wondered if any of those accounts had money in them.

Looking up at us, Maria asked, 'What was the real problem with our sheep?'

'Snails killed 'em,' the Indian flatly stated.

I wanted to correct him, but didn't get a chance. Maria hadn't finished her say. 'Well, honey… after two weeks of time, service and medicines, I'm sure the amount is substantial. So why don't you divide it into thirds and write one check on each bank.'

My head was spinning…what's going on here? Maria just called the Indian 'honey'. Did my uncle forget to tell me that Maria had left her husband John for the ranch's Indian foreman?

Sitting down in the desk's immense swivel chair, Indian Jim began making out the checks for my clinic. While he was signing, I could plainly read the printed name on the top of each, Johnathan James Nogala.

This Indian owned the Mud River Ranch—*he's* Maria's husband. Why didn't I realize it? Feeling my face turn hot and red, I was glad Maria sat behind me and couldn't see my shock. Jim—or actually John—was busy looking over the bill. So, in these next few moments, I needed to quickly gather my wits and focus on what I'd say next.

Composing myself as best I could, I forced a smile when John passed the bank drafts to me. Shaking hands, we acknowledged each other with sincere thanks for the successful completion of a nearly impossible job. He kindly invited me to stay on for dinner. Since my wife was expecting me home that evening, I had an excuse to decline. I really wanted to leave…and sort out my muddled thoughts.

Politely saying my goodbyes, I backed out of the library while tipping my hat toward Maria. Almost on cue, Lobo got up from his sprawled, napping position next to her and walked me to the door. The dog's temperament and skill had been of such great value to me during the past two weeks…I knew I'd miss him. But I didn't think I'd ever see him, John and Maria, or this unusual ranch again."

* * * * *

More than restless, my uncle was ready to hang up…and I didn't think he'd heard a word I'd said. But I decided to finish my story anyway:

"As you know, uncle, I was still skeptical. So I called the banks when I returned home to see if Indian Jim's checks were any good. And, no matter which bank official I spoke to, I received almost the same response. The first officer couldn't stop laughing and thought I'd made a joke. Realizing I was serious, he said I might as well have asked if a check from Donald Trump would bounce. The second executive simply said, 'Jonathan Nogala is the bank's owner and the president of our board of directors.' The third, a young woman, giggled and said, 'I thought everyone knew Indian Jim was the richest man in the state...he's a billionaire.'"

I repeated this 'billionaire' comment to see if my uncle was listening.

"So?...and what time are you obliged to be at his ranch?"

Talking to him was like trying to explain liver flukes to Indian Jim. "I already told you...Maria's bringing the puppy here, instead. How come the two of you never hear anything I say?"

"We hear ya, sonny, we hear ya...but we treat'cha like a kid 'cause ya still got some growin' up to do."

Suddenly becoming serious, he got a little more personal. "You're stuck on how ya think we *should* be...instead of acceptin' us as we are. Ya had your nose out of joint for years just 'cause John wears torn shirts...and he don't match your high 'n mighty idea of what he should look like or wear 'cause he's so rich. All ya need know is Indian Jim's a good man...and hard workin'. He's built everythin' hisself and deserves livin' the way he wants. He don't hav'ta wear fancy shirts...he don't hav'ta be phony. Look at me...I always got on ol' shirts. Money and show...they don't mean nothin', sonny...they ain't what's real."

Feeling a lump come to my throat, I wondered how long he'd wanted to get that off his chest. It was the most he'd ever said to me at one time. And it took me off guard…because he was right. Nothing was said for a few moments…and when I tried to thank him for being honest with me, he shrugged it off and laughed.

"For a snot-nosed kid, you listen good…and my friend John says you're a purdy fair doctor, too."

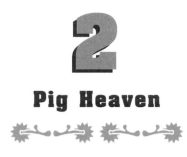

2

Pig Heaven

Sporting a reputation throughout Texas as a brilliant civil engineer, Elvis Fogel had been coming to our clinic for years to occasionally board his pedigreed black Lab, Bogie. When the likable young fellow let it be known he was trying to purchase the old Ramie homestead, I agreed to get him together with Melvin Ramie. A native Texan, and dyed-in-the-wool farmer, Melvin owned over three hundred acres just north and west of the Dallas county line—a prime hunk of real estate.

Proposed and on the drawing boards was an ambitious undertaking, a one-million-square-foot shopping complex. Conceived by Fogel as a 'Shoppers Heaven', the mall would feature only the finest couturiers and high-end retail shops.

I accompanied the soft-spoken Melvin to his first meeting with Fogel at the engineer's lavishly appointed penthouse office. And what unfolded was the kind of scenario I'd only seen in movies. Melvin may have appeared to be a slow-moving plow-boy, but he was nobody's fool—even when matched against Fogel's army of lawyers known for their power games and expertise in corporate politics.

During the formal meeting, Fogel's legal team quickly promised millions of dollars and pulled out contracts ready for Melvin's immediate signature. But Melvin kept on chewing his tobacco…refusing to sign on the dotted line until a comfortable arrangement could be made for his six sows and their piglets.

Fogel, usually known for his cool head, stammered when asking Melvin, " Now, now…do you understand that we're offering you the chance of a lifetime… more money…more than you can ever spend in your retirement?"

The eighty-year-old Melvin was quiet for a moment, then leaned in to spit his chaw in the wastebasket at Fogel's feet. "But, sonny…" he said, "I done been retired for thirty years…and don't need your money."

"You don't need eight million dollars?" Elvis Fogle repeated.

Melvin spat again. "That's a bunch, all right," he said without expression. "But what about my pigs?" he asked, mentioning each one by name. "There's Elsie and Mary Beth…named after my two daughters, 'cause ya know they're both beautiful. Then there's Ima and Youra, Cutie and Gertrude. Ima hog and Youra hog can be temperamental…so they ain't gonna take kindly to movin'. Their waller sits next to the chicken coop, at the dead-center of the property. What do I tell 'em?"

Unable to control his impatience, an overly cynical attorney sputtered, "With eight million dollars, your animals can buy any farm they want—anywhere they want."

"God, they're just pigs…bacon," another member of the legal team laughed.

At that, I sank heavily in my seat. I knew Melvin would sooner slaughter that slick-tongued lawyer before he'd ever eat pork. At the 'bacon' comment, Melvin calmly stood up, slowly stretched his gangly, long legs, and walked to the door. His hulking, six-foot-four presence in the doorway was almost startling. The thin, black-vested attorneys sitting around the boardroom table suddenly seemed dwarfed and pale.

Then turning, and looking for—but not finding—another place to spit his tobacco, Melvin kept chewing without a swallow and quietly said, "Nope, boys. *Ten* million…or my pigs stay in the middle of the property until they die of natural causes."

After a chorus of complaints from the power brokers, the apparent leader of the pack said, "Wait a minute now…we've already offered you more than its worth."

Melvin paused again. "*Thank* so?" Raising the lid of his worn imitation-leather briefcase, he spit his chaw inside—then walked out of the room commenting, "Best you *thank* twice, boys…"

I'd been sitting at the side of the room, with my back to the wall. So when the six lawyers shuffled uncomfortably and whispered comments to one another, I couldn't make out what they were saying.

Elvis Fogel—the only one to smile—broke the silence, "Doc, can you help us out here?"

Somewhat awed by what took place, I simply asked how he thought I could help.

"By movin' those pigs of his to the back part of that land parcel," he explained.

"Gimme a call," I said, figuring Elvis had just accepted Melvin's deal without even talking it over with those attorneys of his. "Y'all agree to give Melvin everything he wants...get the papers signed, sealed, and delivered...then I'll help ya."

* * * * *

A few weeks later, Tracy and Dr. Vest came lurching into Twin Oaks, dripping wet and leaving the trail of two mud ducks. "Darn that Elvis Fogel," Tracy swore, as she chipped flakes of drying black gumbo-soil from her hair. "He's got the brains of a..."

In worse shape than Tracy, Dr. Vest looked like he'd been in a mud-wrestling contest. My partner's sleeves and cuffs were splattered with filth. And the two of them smelled even worse than they looked.

"Geeze," I gasped, "...where have y'all been?"

"Elvis Fogel's and his new Vintage Gate mall," Dr. Vest explained. "We've been movin' those swine of Melvin Ramie's."

"Who got dirtier...you or them?" I teased.

"I don't want to talk about it," Tracy snipped.

"Doc, it was another good idea gone wrong," my partner said. "Let's just say that an engineer should never design a pig waller."

Tracy couldn't help herself and interrupted, "Ah, shucks... here's the nuts and bolts. Elvis called while you were over at Ed's gettin' your hair cut. At his request—since *you* offered to help — we went to the construction site to shoo a few lazy sows from one pen to another. We thought...how hard could that be?"

"Anyway," Tracy continued, "…in the middle of 'bulldozer alley' with earth movers and cranes stirrin' up dust, Mr. Fogel led us to six red sows and a dozen piglets. He…"

Dr. Vest grinned and took up the story, "He pointed toward the new pen. So I backed our stock trailer up to the gate of the old pen. Then we tromped through a six-inch-deep waller of slop to catch piglets on the run."

"It was a scream," Tracy finally laughed.

"Hell," Dr. Vest said, "…they squealed and snorted loud enough for everyone in the county to hear."

Somehow, I knew what was coming—this would all be blamed on me.

My partner held up his hands, covered with dried brown grunge. "Do you see this? Have you any idea how nasty those sows were? This should'a been YOU."

"We had mud flyin' everywhere," Tracy said. "When the pigs were loaded, we drove to the new pen that Elvis's crew had prepared."

Dr. Vest went on, "You should'a seen it…that professionally designed pig run has an adobe shade-hut on one end and a mosaic-tiled pool at the other. There's even redwood decking around the edges, and a misting fountain. Can you believe, a misting fountain? And Elvis must'a put somethin' special in the waller-mud, too, 'cause it's smooth like some ritzy spa. The whole place is a dang resort!"

Shaking with laughter, he tried to continue, "When Elvis opened the trailer, the pig stampede began. The sows ran for the shade of the hut…but the piglets scrambled for the cool mud."

At this point, he and Tracy doubled over, unable to control themselves.

"What?…what?" I pleaded, "What's so funny?"

"One by one," Tracy said, "…each baby pig dove in. And…one by one they each sank."

"That darn waller was four feet deep!" Dr. Vest said. "Those poor little piglets sank faster than rocks in quicksand."

I was horrified, "NO!…what did y'all do?"

"We went PIG BOBBIN'—that's what we did. We moved faster than we've ever moved…and one by one, leg by leg, and tail by nose, we pulled 'em all out," said Tracy. "That's why Dr. Vest has mud in his ears. And that's why them sows and piggies are now back in their old pen."

"Yep," Dr. Vest snapped, "…and next time, *you* get to move 'em."

"Me?" I asked, pretending to be surprised.

"Nope…the three of you. You, Elvis, and Melvin…it was your deal all along," he added.

As he walked over to the sink to wash up, my partner seemed to be reading my mind when he emphatically said, "And Doc, you best not be goin' anywhere 'til this is all settled."

When Elvis finished the needed changes—and had drained the depths of the new waller, I went over to help. Then, when all was ready—like ducklings behind Mother Goose—the cute little pigs followed the lead sow, Gertrude, to their new pen. Elsie, the oldest sow, had been trained by Melvin to go on walks, and just needed a leash. Finally calm and settled into their new home at the rear of the mall property, the swine basked on the sundeck of their patio, while the 'piggly-wigglies' splashed around in their shallow 'spa'. With a sigh of relief, I felt the situation was well in hand; but there was still one turn of events that none of us, especially Fogel, could have anticipated.

Since the engineer enjoyed such a high profile, the media had him under constant scrutiny. It didn't take long for the papers and television to create all kinds of coverage for this story, along with the expected cartoons and jokes. While the whole comical episode was becoming the talk of the town, Fogel's thirty-million-dollar 'elite' mall was dubbed 'Piglet Outlet'…a name that stuck. The irony was never lost on Elvis.

During and after the grand opening of the complex, nearly everyone coming to the mall stopped to visit the pigs in their fancy haven. They would first gather there to socialize, before strolling on to do their shopping. It was becoming the 'in' thing to do.

Ultimately, everyone got what they wanted: Melvin became a kind of 'Grandpa' to the many visiting children—letting them take turns walking Elsie around on her leash. Touched by all the attention, the amiable farmer made an appearance at the waller at least three or four times a week. His pigs were thriving and becoming local celebrities, of sorts. There wasn't anyone who didn't know each one by name.

We thought Fogel and his investors would never get over the embarrassment of feeling personally insulted by the 'Piglet Outlet' tag for their grand mall. But once Vintage Gate became a permanent attraction, with tourists arriving daily, they eventually adjusted to the disappointment and—as the saying goes, '…cried all the way to the bank.'

3

Late in the Day

eliveries are accepted at the back of the building," snapped the valet as he approached my truck.

Ignoring the young man, I simply gave him a cordial nod and handed him the keys to the battle-weary Ol' Blue. Then grabbing my medicine bag and jumping out, I headed toward the lobby of the classy and exclusive Turtle Creek town-homes of Palace Court.

Expansive rose gardens blanketed the surrounding terrain, extending to over 300 acres devoted to play and leisure-time activities. There were golf courses, tennis courts, swimming pools, jogging trails, and riding stables. This was definitely an ultra-posh home for only a wealthy few.

I'd come straight from the pastures…and looked it. After castrating colts and branding cows for most of the day, I'm sure my worn, dirty coveralls had a distinctive smell, as well.

Looking me up and down, the unsmiling, tuxedo-clad doorman raised his white-gloved hand to signal 'stop'. "You can't go in there, Sir."

In no mood to debate, I strutted on in. The bewildered gent—doing his job well—pretended to be polite. "And who, Sir, may I ask…has requested your presence?"

Glancing over my shoulder to reply, I gave him a nonchalant reply, "Your boss, Linda Hanna…she owns these fancy diggin's."

Obviously worried about the presence of a surly cowboy, the conscientious doorman followed on my heels as I punched the elevator button. "May I ring her suite, Sir…and announce your arrival?"

"If you want to be wasting your time…Linda's still on the top floor?"

The gold-leaf doors of the mirrored lift closed before he could answer, and I soared upward toward the ninth floor.

Stepping out into the 'receiving foyer'…a breathy, recorded voice greeted me, "Welcome to the home of Linda Hanna." English tapestries and oil paintings of British lords and ladies covered the walls of the long hallway. Ornate furnishings, presumably from an ancient Scottish castle, adorned the entire entrance. And massive floor-to-ceiling glass panels at each end provided spectacular views of the city skyline.

At first, I wondered where an overwhelming, sweet scent was coming from, and thought it might be incense. Then I saw the dozens and dozens of tall crystal vases, each crowded with fresh-cut red roses.

Whenever I came to this place, I ended up shaking my head at the odd rags-to-riches story behind the 'lady of the house'.

Linda was really *Boom-Boom* Lindy Lee...the one-time notorious 'madame' of Dallas county.

The only real part of Linda was her surname, Lee. She was, indeed, a distant relative to the Confederate General Robert E. Lee. The rest was all phony, except for the inherited money from her deceased husband, Blanton Hanna. He had acquired his fortune in a number of shady businesses, and owned almost every other topless strip-joint in Texas. He first met Linda at one of those hot spots. Popular for her unique rendition of slowly unraveling herself from a Rebel flag...Linda became Blanton's favorite dancer.

When police discovered that one of his companies was being used as a cover to launder bad money, Blanton ended up serving a short stint in prison. During this time, Linda tried to become respectable by going into the real estate business and doing well at it. Unfortunately, some of her husband's old dealings must have caught up with him. Two years back, he was accidentally killed in one of his own bars when an argument with a former colleague escalated to a vicious brawl with broken beer bottles.

Though she was as brash and ostentatious as the bubbling, gold Cupid fountain in her foyer, I still couldn't fault Linda's current lifestyle. And I watched in amusement as she swung open the doors and rushed to embrace me—her sentences running together as usual. "Hey, Doc...dang it, but it's good to see ya. But I've been as fretful as a French whore without a man, worryin' about Chester and Dixie." Framed photos of the two strays—Chester, a mixed-breed terrier, and Dixie, her adopted orange and white alley cat—were always kept in the center of her lengthy Victorian mantelpiece.

I was taken aback by the way Linda looked. She'd had a few facelifts in the past. But her complexion was now fish-belly white, and the paleness only accentuated the lizard tightness of the current lift—or maybe it was a chemical peel. A fluorescent-pink, feathered robe hung loosely around her still-ample body, draping down to her silk, heeled slippers. And despite the fact that she had next to nothing on, she still managed to wear her diamond bracelets. Trying hard to remain glamorous with heavy makeup and rouge, the lady was the picture of a once-famous—but still spirited—flamboyant actress.

Winking at Linda and her beckoning finger, I followed her into the living room. The antique furniture was covered with floral sheets for Dixie and Chester's comfort. But the home appeared ransacked, with two broken lamps on the floor, shattered wine goblets, and a foot-long crack in the balcony's sliding glass door.

"Linda, what happened here? Have you been robbed?"

Shaking her dyed-blond curls from side to side, she pointed toward the utility room. There were her depressed pets, enclosed behind the gate of a baby pen. Chester, lying flat on his stomach with his tail straight out behind him, didn't even look up at me. And Dixie sat quietly in the corner, her eyes lowered. Linda must have just scolded them.

I laughed at the destructive culprits, "It looks like y'all are in big trouble."

"Doc, I'm afraid Chester's jaw is broken." In fact, that's what she'd said in the emergency message that got me out here so late in the day. But the terrier didn't appear to have a fracture. Chester's right eye was swollen shut, and the jowl on the same side of his face was thick and sagging. He didn't whimper in pain when I put pressure on the swollen area. In fact, the little dog looked more guilty than hurt.

Linda went on, "…and if that ain't gross enough, Dixie's limpin' on a bum front leg."

Her cat hobbled toward me when I took down the toddler-gate. Though in obvious discomfort, she purred while extending her paw. Again, there was no fracture. Dixie's forearm was sore and the swollen tissues enlarged her foot. I was beginning to realize only one thing could account for these problems.

"Chester, come here, boy," I said. Petting and comforting him, I took his muzzle in my hands and spread his fattened lips apart.

This surprised Linda. "Doc, what in blazes are you lookin' for?"

"…a stinger," I replied, as I quickly plucked a tiny, brown splinter from the inside of Chester's upper lip. It now made sense as to what caused such havoc in Linda's home.

"Linda, your lovely place is crammed with fresh flowers of every kind. And there's a common denominator here between fresh flowers and pollen…bees and bee stings! That's what's ailing your pets. See the puffed up, swollen spots where they've been stung? Dixie must have swatted one with her paw, and Chester probably snapped one out of the air, as dogs often do. The rest we can only imagine. But the likelihood is that Dixie was wildly chasing a couple of flying wasps, and the dog was following in pursuit. After racing over counters, between lamp-stands, and across furniture, they finally smacked headlong into the plate-glass door…getting stung during the process."

Giving the little cohorts-in-crime antihistamine and cortisone injections to resolve any inflammatory allergic reactions,

I left a few necessary pills so Linda could administer them the next day.

"And, Boom Boom...I have something else I want you to do." I enjoyed calling Linda by her former stage name...it always seemed to flatter her. "I'm giving you this can of bug repellent. After I leave, spray it around each room and in the foyer where you have all those roses. And be sure to tell your gardener to check for any bugs or bees on future bouquets before he brings them inside. Okay?"

As I was about to leave the alley cat, retired stripper, and stray mutt in the contentment of their opulent environment, Linda said, "Oh, Doc, you're a regular genius...and always there for me. Will my babies be all right now?"

"Don't worry about them, they'll be just fine," I said as I walked out the ambassador doors, making a mock bow before one of the portraits of a British lord. "See ya later, Lindy Lee, it's been fun..."

Sprinting out through the lobby, in a much better mood than when I came in, I encountered the same doorman. Relieved to see me departing, he asked, "Sir, does the young man know which car is yours?"

"It's the only truck in the parking lot...big, blue 'n dented," I laughed.

Purposely gunning the motor and peeling away, I'm sure Ol' Blue left dark and muddy skid-marks on the Palace Court's yellow stone driveway. This wasn't very nice of me. But it was the end of a long, long day...and engaging in such a youthful display simply made me feel a whole lot better.

Heart of a Winner

Sam never sounded like this before. Preparing for dinner when I took his emergency call...the anger and sadness in his shaking voice sent chills down my spine. Overwhelmed with emotion, his words tumbled together...as he tried telling me his Quarter horse stallion had just been hit by a three-ton truck.

A magnificent racehorse, Ultra-Light Dash was not only fast and beautiful—but worth more than any other horse in the state. Having won three out of his last four races, he was the celebrated star of the internationally known Stride Farms, just five miles from our home. And Sam Hoffman was the long-time foreman of this two-thousand-acre equestrian breeding and racing facility.

Struggling to explain, Sam's voice broke, "Doc...two fellas tried to steal Dash...but in getting away from them, Dash crashed through the fence, ran across the road...and in this thick fog, he was...."

I couldn't wait to hear any more. Dropping the receiver, I turned and bolted out the door without saying anything to Karen or my son.

The screen door creaked and slammed shut behind me. The coolness of the damp night air hit my cheeks as I frantically searched the porch for a pair of boots. Several feet of dense, gray fog hugged the ground. Only the tops of my boots could be seen when I grabbed them and scrambled toward Ol' Blue. Smoky wet clouds layered the earth in every direction. Looking like it was smack-dab in the middle of a pond, Ol' Blue's hood was the only thing visible. In my rush, I kept stumbling—with one boot on and the other in hand—stubbing my toe twice before managing to get into the cab.

This attempted kidnapping was a serious situation. It may be different elsewhere. But in Texas, horse stealing is still a capital offense. And getting the animal hurt in the process was unthinkable. "Hell, some laws ain't never need be changed," my dad would say, "...it's a simple fact of life...and don't matter if it's an ol' plow pony or a racing stud...no one messes with another person's horse."

I didn't need pavement beneath my tires to go flying in the direction of the stables. Ol' Blue fishtailed and banked around the familiar S-shaped curves. Hearing loose gravel slapping the wheel-wells, I knew I'd gone away from the centerline, and was getting close to the ditch. Karen's parting words of "...please drive slowly in this soupy weather," echoed in my ears. Gripping the steering wheel tighter and tighter, I maneuvered Ol' Blue further into the fog. My headlights finally bounced from the ground-clouds to illuminate the iron-arched entrance to Stride Farms.

Sam would be waiting for me at the stallion barn. Ol' Blue's hubs straddled the horizontal pipes of the cattle guard, and I aimed for the only lights in sight. Barely making out Sam's lean silhouette in the doorway, I did see an unmistakable shape of a rifle lying in the crook of his folded arms. The shadow of his tiny wife, Susan, was behind him—pacing back and forth.

Sliding to a stop and leaping from Ol' Blue, I asked, "Susan, Sam...how bad is it?"

"Come see for yourself, Doc," they murmured together.

In the center stall—in a state of shock—was Ultra-Light Dash...still standing. Pools of blood were under each hoof. I opened the latch and reached for the dangling cotton lead rope to gently guide the injured horse into more light. I didn't know where to begin. And I knew by the glaze in his eyes that he was standing by shear guts alone. But he was bearing weight on all four limbs, so none of his legs were broken...a miracle, I thought.

Turning to fetch what was needed, Sam held on to the blood-soaked halter to keep Dash still. I rummaged through my medicine box praying I had volumes and volumes of thread, while Susan—who usually had Sam do all the talking—began filling me in on the details. "When we heard the commotion behind the barn, Sam ran out in the dark, and took a shot at the thieves. On the road, two guys in a tanker-truck were on their way to work the night shift at the plastics plant. They couldn't see Dash in the fog...until it was too late."

Needing to concentrate, I rapidly checked what I had: tranquilizer, painkiller, and anti-inflammatory medicines. Talking to myself, I inventoried, "...I.V. catheter, thread, suture pack, and fluids, fluids, and more fluids. Thread, thread, and more thread…bandages, gauze and tape."

Susan felt the need to keep talking. "Dash must've jumped like a deer in their headlights. By the looks of the hood and roof of the truck, he must've rolled like a boulder over the dashboard. How both men coulda' survived is beyond me. Dash must weigh fifteen hundred pounds. Ya know, Doc…he's built like a brick wall."

With Susan helping me, and our arms full, we carried all the medical supplies into the barn. I was still wondering about the two guys and the truck, when she explained, "They've gone to the hospital in Sam's pickup. One man was asleep at the time of the wreck. He was slump't in the front seat… and is okay. The other has a bad gash on the top of his head where the roof caved in on 'im…but don't know if it was from Dash or when they lost control and went down the embankment. These guys were real shook up when they came up to the barn to tell Sam about Dash." Looking out into the depths of the fog as if I could see anything, she added, "See there? Their truck careened to the bottom of the old creek bed…and it's still there."

Dash was in the worst shape possible. In the dim light, between the seams of Sam's hasty, makeshift bandages, blood seeped from the covered lacerations. Quickly administering necessary medications to ease the sorrel's discomfort, I began working on the largest cuts first. After plucking hundreds of pieces of shattered glass from his flesh, and stitching multiple skin tears on his face, neck and chest, I knelt down to begin unwrapping his forelegs—only to discover more torn tissues than I'd ever seen on a standing animal. Gravel, dirt, metal, grass, plastic, and chunks of the never-ending glass filled the raw spaces that his skin once covered.

At the sight, Sam staggered back—and his breaths became short. During the confusion, he hadn't realized the full severity of Dash's injuries. The skin above the stallion's right knee was rolled like a sock down to his ankle. His forearm was hanging on to the bone by only tangled strips of frayed muscle fibers and exposed tendons. Under the bruised skin on his lower chest was the blade of a windshield-wiper wedged into the subcutaneous layers of tissue. Blood was puddling beneath my soles, as Susan began unwrapping the other front leg. When I turned to lay the saturated bandages away from my field of vision, Sam quickly grasped my arm to let me know the left leg was hurt worse than the right.

Kneeling down, I could feel my hair getting soaked from a pumping blood vessel on Dash's side. Sam's hand touched my shoulder as I stood to clamp the leaking vein. "Doc..?" he murmured, "...do ya think we...need to put him to sleep?"

The veteran horseman's hands were trembling when Susan took away the rifle. I shook my head. "No, Sam...nothing appears to be broken, and the tendons and muscles are somewhat intact. I think I can save him—if given the chance."

After a long moment, Sam haltingly said, "Then...do whatcha can, Doc..."

Piece by piece—I continued to sew on the massive puzzle that held Dash together. One hour...three...then, four hours passed. Flushing the wounds with antibiotics, the number of sutures needed turned into more than I could count.

Progressing from the four-year-old stud's muzzle to his rump, my fingers, thighs, and back muscles cramped with the tedious assembly of damaged parts. A long slice down the top of Dash's tail would be the last of the many closures performed.

The once handsome horse resembled a mummy. By the time I was done, Dash was wrapped, sprayed, and tied from end to end. My joints creaked as I stood back to view my work.

Slowly leading Dash back to his stall, just a few yards away, I mumbled to Sam, "I'll be seein' ya'll tomorrow and tomorrow and tomorrow. All I can say is…I hope they catch those sonny-beetchin' thieves."

"Me, too," Sam said quietly.

We both acknowledged what was ahead of us: dozens and dozens of bandage changes would be required to continually dress the healing wounds—before yards of suture materials could be removed, one knot at a time.

Dash received constant care. But the heart, stamina and will of this remarkable animal was beyond anything we'd ever seen. In less than the two-month recommended rest period, the stallion was back on a training schedule—though gradually at first. He impressed everyone with his progress. And his enormous appetite was a sure sign this champion was regaining his total health.

* * * * *

For weeks on end, I'd been over at the stables with Dash…and my family rarely saw me at dinner. From now on, barring any more emergencies, I'd be there. Walking into our kitchen and hanging my hat on our high-back pine chair, I finally took my place at the supper table. My son only said what he always says, "I'm starving."

Thoroughly exhausted—I didn't say anything. Instead, resting my arms on the inviting table, I was content to take in the wonderful aromas. On this particular night, there'd be a special event. Something was also special about the cooking smells. Karen had prepared all my favorites: chicken-fried steak, mashed potatoes, cream gravy, green beans—and jalapeño cornbread. As I passed my son a plate, Karen asked, "What about grace tonight?"

K.C. put down his fork, and we bowed our heads as he started his prayer. "Thanks, God," he said. A long silence followed, while Karen and I waited. Wondering if that was all he had to say, we looked up as K.C. spoke again. "Oh, and God...help Dash win the race tonight."

"Amen to that!" Karen and I sang out together, as my nine-year-old son snatched a piece of cornbread from between my fingers. Karen reached for the remote so we could watch Ultra-Light Dash's first television debut since the accident.

"There...there he is," I said, pointing to the line of horses being readied at the starting gate. "The big sorrel stallion in the center. Gawd, I hope it ain't too soon for him to be doin' this."

"Which stallion?" Karen asked.

Excitedly pointing again, I said, "There...right there...the one with the scar on his chest...which you probably can't see from here."

Hurriedly pushing back our chairs—forgetting about dinner—the three of us began jumping up and down as the gates opened and Dash sailed into the lead. "Wow, that horse is too much!" K.C. yelled.

Winning by a length, Dash was truly back in full form. As we spotted Susan walking a few steps behind a beaming Sam when they took their place in the Winners' Circle, Karen breathlessly said, "Who could've believed this? By the way, were those kidnappers ever caught?"

Reeling from Dash's phenomenal comeback, I just mumbled under my breath, "Not yet, but when they do, I'll…" Changing the subject, I was still ecstatic, "Ya know, in my mind, this wasn't a race against other horses…Dash's real win was against impossible odds he'd even race again!"

Our dinner was cold by the time we finally settled down to eat…but it was still the best meal I'd ever had.

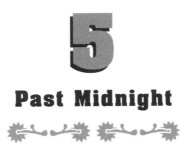

Past Midnight

There are those people who love working nights. And my niece, Sandy, was one of them. Thrilled to take on this duty for our clinic's answering service, she not only enjoyed it—but also looked forward to earning all the extra cash every college freshman seems to crave.

On her third night, at 4:20 A.M. to be exact, the normally cheerful girl called a bit apologetic. "Uncle Doc, I'm so sorry, I know it's still the middle of the night, but there's a frantic woman on the line who says she needs to speak to you right away. It's a Mrs. Hart from Duncanville.

In my half-sleep, I grumbled, "Who? I don't know a Mrs. Hart."

Seemingly anxious to get off the line, Sandy quickly gave me the number and added, "The lady said you'd know all about it."

Duncanville was a long way from Dallas—so I couldn't imagine who it could be. With Karen still asleep at my side, I drowsily dialed the number scrawled on my nightstand memo.

Before I could finish identifying myself, Mrs. Hart began her breathless explanation. "Doc, I'm afraid there's something terribly wrong. When I woke earlier than usual, I immediately noticed blood on everything. It has stopped for now—but I'm worried sick."

"Wait a minute," I blurted, "...who's bleeding, and from where?" She could have been talking about a hamster or a horse.

Agitated, her words tumbled out rapidly, "What do you mean, Doctor? I was in your office last week for a D and C. And you told me to call if I had problems. Now there are small spots of blood all over my bed. You said I might even need a hysterectomy."

This was definitely not my usual wake-up call. Gracefully trying to end our conversation, I said, "Ma'am, I'm afraid you've got the wrong doctor. I'm just a general practitioner...and I don't do that procedure. Besides, I'm..."

Mrs. Hart interrupted, "This isn't Dr. Collerson?"

"No, ma'am, I'm not Dr. Collerson...I'm a..."

Continuing on as though she hadn't heard, the lady from Duncanville said, "Well, maybe you can still help me—I've never had so many problems." Without pausing, she went into detailed explanations of her current malady, including descriptions of her sexual habits. As she began elaborating on her family's history and her daughter's divorce, I finally managed to get a word in edgewise...firmly giving her the reasons why she needed to call her regular physician. At this point—after she'd poured out her woes—I didn't have the heart to tell her I was an animal doctor, and that all my patients had whiskers and tails.

But the lady just couldn't stop jabbering. "Oh, my doctor is nice…but I really like your bedside manner. That's important to me. And besides, Dr. Collerson's probably not up yet."

Realizing the polite approach was getting me nowhere, I almost shouted, "Mrs. Hart, you do need to call your gynecologist as soon as possible!"

"But I want you to be my doctor," she insisted. "You have a nice voice. I'm forty years old. I pay my bills…and I'd be a good patient."

Exasperated, I loudly repeated, "No, ma'am, no…you must call Dr. Collerson—and right away!"

Reluctantly agreeing with me, Mrs. Hart hung up. I couldn't help but imagine how embarrassed she would have been if she had realized I was a vet. I'd been tempted to say, "Come to the clinic, take off your flea collar, and don't hiss at me." I buried my head in the pillow, trying not to laugh.

Karen had awakened…and, mumbling with both eyes closed, asked whom I was talking to.

"Just a lady with reproductive problems," I said.

"Dog or cat?" she asked.

"Neither."

"That's nice," she responded sleepily as she snuggled back under the covers.

★ ★ ★ ★ ★

The story was too good not to tell everyone about it the next morning. And I called my niece first, thinking it wise to spend a little more time training her—especially on ways to screen callers before patching them through to either Dr. Vest or me. In her usual preoccupied state, she didn't seem to take it all that seriously. Though she must have heard me because, after that night, she did her best in weeding out the inappropriate calls.

When I related the night's 'emergency' call to my partner, he began giggling so much he could hardly tell me about the call he once got in the middle of the night. It had been from Lester Agnew, a prominent cattle rancher whom we all knew well.

"Lester called me a while back. It must have been well after midnight. At first he talked about his cow with 'foot-rot'. Then, somehow, he changed the subject to hemorrhoids." Still chuckling, my partner wiped his watering eyes and went on.

"I was even more confused when Lester said, 'Doc, Yankees are like hemorrhoids…they'll come down south, but they won't go back up north.' Well…Lester hem-hawed around, but he finally asked me if his cow's mastitis ointment, prescribed for her udder inflammation, would work on humans, too. He wanted to use it on himself! How was I to respond to that? I insisted he call his personal physician…just as you did with Mrs. Hart."

I started laughing, too, even though I didn't know why.

Regaining his composure, Rich continued his story. "Lester called me back again the next night to say he'd apparently grabbed the wrong tube. And he wanted to know how to get rubber cement…out from between his cheeks!"

"No!" I gasped, "What did you say?"

Dr. Vest held his ribs as though his sides hurt from all the laughing, and sputtered, "I said, 'Call your regular doctor. Hell, Lester, I don't know nothin' 'bout no Yankees'."

Rich and I were both inflicted with the same silly sense of humor. But it was obvious...we were the only two who had fun swapping these 'you-had-to-be-there' moments. Tracy used to roll her eyes and say we were like a couple of kids. That was it, I guess...but I really didn't mind...because it had to be all the laughing that made the long days short—and our partnership strong.

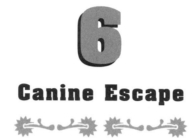

Canine Escape

This was a big deal—our second clinic. Meticulous planning and frayed tempers were paying off as we watched the structural framing of Meadow Creek slowly take shape. Just twenty miles away, the sprawling area of family homes in Flower Mound needed an animal hospital—and we figured it might be time to branch out. A second clinic would give us an unheard-of luxury—backup support.

It wasn't easy. Between regular appointments and ranch calls, little time was left for interviewing prospective vets and administrative staff. I'd already had mixed feelings about this commitment to expand. Adding to my stress-overload was something no one knew about, except my family. I'd received an offer to accept a lucrative position with a national pharmaceutical firm on the east coast. The pros and cons of envisioning such a big change were weighing on my mind. The new spot promised more 'perks' than this Texas boy could imagine—including summer meetings at the home office in Hawaii. Still…I couldn't decide.

Twin Oaks was managing well, but not flourishing. Pre-occupied with this thought and our budget problems, it seemed I surprised a visiting friend when he asked why my jeans were so worn at the knees. "From begging clients to pay their bills," I replied.

For the first time in my practice, I dreaded the beginning of spring roundups—and hoped our new staff at Meadow Creek would be able to take turns with us in handling this seasonal responsibility. Already on a deadline to vaccinate and de-worm three thousand head of horses, artificially breed the mares, and castrate the calf herds…my worry must have been obvious.

"Don'tcha fret none, Doc," Tracy said, "…we'll get 'em done…like always." I greatly admired the optimism of this pony-tailed wonder…and couldn't imagine any day without her.

After backing up Ol' Blue behind Twin Oaks, we opened the rear doors leading through the kennels to the supply room. The vast amount of medicines and supplies needed for the roundups had been shipped and inventoried two months earlier. All we had to do was get it loaded and administered. Dr. Vest pulled his rig into place alongside mine. And we began rushing in and out of the clinic with armloads of equipment to outfit each truck.

Involved with the job at hand, everyone dismissed the usual sounds coming from the boarding kennels…until one alarm stood out. Billy, our kennel boy, yelled, "LOOK OUT!" as he careened past us. Tracy jumped to the side, and I flinched as a little dog whizzed by. It was 'Annie', who often stayed with us whenever her owner was out of town. But now the pup was loose and barreling for safety.

"Catch 'er!" shouted Billy.

Tracy grabbed for the escaping corgi's non-existent tail, then scrambled on her knees trying to grasp a handful of fur. She screamed as Annie nipped at her ankle before zigzagging between my legs and darting for the wide-open spaces. Neither of us could capture the little cylinder on pegs. Her collar was off…and she had twisted and squirmed through everyone's fingers. Dr. Vest tried to corner the tan and white flash, but failed, too. Annie was free. She had jumped from the bathtub and, still covered with suds, sprinted past us all with her paws clawing toward the horizon. Billy's shouts were still ringing in our ears.

"Don't let her get away," Dr. Vest hollered.

"Holy sh…." Tracy blurted, pounding her fist on the pavement.

Running in hot pursuit, as if any of us could run as fast as a dog being chased, I commanded, "Come 'ere, you slippery critter." I yelled again as Annie bolted under a truck parked across the street.

Geeze, I thought, how will I explain this to her owner? I didn't take my eyes off of her…silently praying she wouldn't get struck by a car. Annie's ears were flat, and her stubby legs were churning away as soap billowed off her back in small, bubbly clouds. She began weaving between rolling cars. Billy's long strides passed mine, and I choked, "Git 'er!"

Having dashed for the first few hundred yards, I stumbled and slowed to a trot. All I could see was the back of Billy's green shirt and his curly red hair, bobbing up and down, over car hoods and around trunks—then Annie's broad rump racing around the bumper of a black Ford. Our agile kennel boy, proving his local track star status, seemed to be everywhere at once, jumping over bushes, around curb posts—and finally dropping to his knees in order to spot Annie scooting under floorboards and circling tires of parked vehicles.

Barking all the while, Annie let Billy know when he was getting too close. She taunted him into chasing her around and around the dentist's office facing our clinic. Then she squinted her eyes, pointed her nose, and sprinted toward the busiest intersection in Dallas. I froze. On a dead run, Dr. Vest tried to cut her off, waving his arms and yelling, "YAA…YAA!" He shouted to me that she was coming my way.

"There!" Tracy yelled, as Annie suddenly reversed her direction and blasted between us in a blurring streak of whiskers, slobber, and paws. Back across the street and down the alley she trotted, appearing cocky and proud of herself. I called out hoping to appeal to her, "Here Annie…." Surprised, she stopped and turned. Then wagging her butt and panting, she dared me to chase her further. At least she's not frantic, I thought.

Billy joined me in the alley blockade. And as soon as Dr. Vest appeared, we formed a human fence. There was one car parked behind the beauty salon—and no way out for Annie. "We've got 'er…slow and easy," I said, "…no sudden moves. We don't want to crowd her."

Annie hesitated, then hunkered down when she saw Dr. Vest. Her head twisted from side to side, as she'd watch me, Dr. Vest, then me again. Searching for a way out, she inched along on her stomach under a parked yellow Buick.

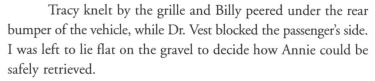
Tracy knelt by the grille and Billy peered under the rear bumper of the vehicle, while Dr. Vest blocked the passenger's side. I was left to lie flat on the gravel to decide how Annie could be safely retrieved.

"Can you reach her, Billy?" I asked.

"I'm not stickin' my hand under there," he replied.

Annie was out of our reach, centered in the middle of the car. She was just lying there with that endearing expression on her face. But we knew she could and would bite. Crawling, face-to-face, into her confined territory wasn't the best idea.

"SHOO!..." Billy said. But he was in no position to be issuing orders. Annie growled and her sudden glare was a warning.

For some reason, I felt my whole career was balancing on our next move. We considered the clinic's catch-pole as an emergency option, but agreed it would be too traumatic for her.

"Everybody...come with me," I said. Standing and turning, I started to walk away. Dr. Vest, Billy, and Tracy looked at me in disbelief—but they followed. "Don't look back," I said, as we continued to walk. "Annie, c'mon...c'mon girl."

She would either bolt or she would follow us. It was hot under the car, but she didn't budge. Beginning to think I'd made the wrong decision, I caught a glimpse of Annie starting to crawl out from under the old Buick. She whimpered as if to say...*where are y'all going?* After one muffled bark, she stood and slowly moved ten yards in our direction.

"Tracy, peel away from the group," I said softly. "Make a big circle—and get between Annie and that car."

Annie ventured further and further from her chosen refuge. "Y'all keep on walking," I said. "Don't turn around."

Now alone, I sat down in the alley with my back turned
to Annie. Not wanting my body to show any signs of aggression,
or even interest, I sat Indian-style and motionless with my arms
and legs folded. Annie stopped several feet behind me and lay
down—with her chin resting on her front paws. Her eyes shifted
between the retreating Tracy and me, as though she was trying
to decide which one she could trust. I quietly asked Tracy to
throw a handful of gravel at the nearby dumpster.

At the sight of Tracy's swinging arm, Annie came flying
toward me...with the patter of her pads making clicking sounds
across the loose, pebbly gravel. Sticking her cold, wet nose under
my elbow, she wormed her muddy, warm body into my lap. Both
ends of her chubby torso wiggled. Her breath smelled worse than
the aroma from the dumpster. And her long tongue lapped and
slurped all over my cheek—but I didn't mind.

I fell on my back with Annie on my chest. She barked
with glee as I cuddled her and lifted her round body away from
my face. "You little butterball...where were you going? You scared
us to death."

Never one to waste a moment of time, Tracy brought us
back to reality with a firm reminder of our need to get on the
road. Our jaunt with Annie had put us behind schedule.

At that moment, through the back door walked Dr. Bill
Horton and Dr. Seth Ward, the young vets interested in eventually joining us when the new clinic was up and running. They
agreed to be our relief team at Twin Oaks for the next few weeks,
since we'd be away handling the roundups and breeding pro-
grams. This would be the perfect opportunity for both doctors
to get acquainted with our clients and our unique practice—since

critters under our care were not only the small pets in town—but also the horses and farm animals in the surrounding countryside.

"You're late," Tracy said, passing them by with bundles of supplies in her arms.

Seth and Bill knew nothing of the details of our 'track meet' with Jackie Berdwall's corgi. And Billy tried to explain why we were all out of breath and covered with dirt.

Exhausted from her morning marathon of leading three so-called professionals through the streets of Dallas, Annie obliged Billy by letting him give her a relaxing, no-hassle bath. Then she took a three-hour snooze before Jackie came in to pick her up. By that time, the three of us were already on the road.

Lucky for us, Billy held down the fort. When it came to tact and charm, he beat us all. Whatever he said must have worked…because he told us Annie's owner wasn't upset and didn't appear surprised at her pup's truant behavior. For the past six years, she and her two teenage girls had been raising corgis for a living on their small farm north of Dallas. Apparently, our episode was mild compared to most antics she'd seen. Knowing Billy was hoping to become a vet, she filled him in on the peculiarities of the breed—and said she loved corgis, but, "As y'all have seen, they're smart and a whole lot of fun, but they're incorrigible…and their stubborn streak always gets 'em into a whole mess of trouble."

A week later, Seth called us during roundups to say a super-sized box of chocolates just arrived at the clinic with a note from Jackie expressing her appreciation, as well as her surprise, that all four of us had worked so hard in safely bringing in her clever 'escapee'.

This seemingly inconspicuous, 'everyday' event only increased my indecision on whether I'd continue practicing or not. I kept reminding myself, over and over...the other job offer was all about 'corporate' business. And I had to admit...I was all about 'people' business. I liked the folks here in the community. Everyone knew us—and depended on us. Most Texas towns were growing faster than you could blink, and ours was no different. Yet I felt we'd never lose our 'small town' country values. Somehow... I had a difficult time imagining Chicago in quite the same way.

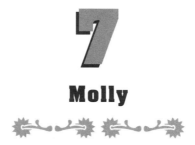

Molly

It all started so innocently—on Sunday, a day of rest. Karen and K.C. had taken their seats next to me in church. Feeling someone's hot breath on the back of my neck made me turn around. Fred Landsberry, leaning forward in the pew directly behind me, tapped me on the shoulder, whispering, "Doc, will you spay and declaw my cat?"

"Sure," I whispered back, as our pastor began walking toward the lectern.

"But, Doc, this isn't your average alley cat," he said, with some hesitation. By this time, my favorite preacher, Jim Foley, had started his sermon.

I grabbed my hymnal to write a quick, penciled note to Fred on the inside front cover: *What do you mean? You know I've done a thousand of these, including your two raccoons and the hedgehog. So how difficult can it be? Bring her to the clinic tomorrow,*

Monday, I'll do it then. After passing the book over my shoulder to Fred, I waited.

Nearing the end of our service, as the congregation began lustily singing 'How Great Thou Art', Fred tapped me again to say, "Doc, it might be Friday…'cause we're shippin' 'er in. Are ya *sure* about this?"

"I'm sure," I said, a little too loudly. Karen elbowed me sharply. "Y'all hush!" Grinning from ear to ear, my son covered his mouth to muffle his snickering. He lived for moments like this, when his mother scolded me instead of him.

I turned around, but Fred was already walking out the side entrance. No point in catching up with him, I thought. I'd be seeing him soon enough.

This was a man I greatly admired—for many reasons. Landsberry was the best horse trainer around. In fact, he could train any creature to do just about anything. Time after time, we felt privileged to witness his unusual talents. Even difficult animals—those others had given up on—would submit to his spell. Perhaps it was his phenomenal patience, or his lack of fear. Or maybe he learned some secret from the local Indian shamans; he'd spent a lot of time with them over the years. I told Dr. Vest he might exude some kind of domesticating pheromone not yet discovered. But my partner thought I was too lenient in continually encouraging Fred's need to adopt every stray he heard about. All the same, I felt proud to be part of the man's network to save as many animals as possible—no matter what the circumstances were.

Near Celina, Fred's immense farm was home to sixty spotted Kiowa ponies, two yellow Manx house cats, a lion called

'Maxine', a dozen raccoons, and an elephant, 'Polly'. There were a couple of dozen other critters, too, including an egg-bound emu. I didn't know emus could have the same malady as other birds—so Fred patiently supervised the treatment, helping to further my avian training. I realized then...he had as much medical knowledge as any vet.

The trainer had everyone's respect—and deservedly so. Though not an imposing physical figure, it didn't matter. On the slight side, five-foot-six and a little balding, he had what no one else had: a warming calmness about him that held both man and beast captive—in a most positive way.

By the time Friday evening rolled around, I still hadn't heard from him. His younger brother finally called me at home explaining, "Doc, this is Barry. There was a flight delay coming in from Seattle, and I've just arrived at Dallas-Fort Worth International Airport with the mountain lion. Fred wants you to..."

"WHAT?" I interrupted Barry in mid-sentence. My mouth dropped open, and all I could do was repeat myself. "WHAT? Put Fred on the phone right away..."

Pausing for a moment, Barry said, "I can't...Fred and Molly, the cougar, just left. They're on their way to your place right now."

I told Karen I'd be rushing over to the clinic to meet Fred and 'Molly', and hoped I could put a stop to this. With a light peck on the cheek, resembling a kiss for someone on death row, she said, "Goodbye, sweetheart...don't let Molly get her claws into you."

It was evident someone had let the word out. Pulling up to the hospital, I noticed two vans and an SUV parked in front of Fred's Dodge Ram. Tracy's pickup was also parked around back. My ever-thoughtful wife thought to let our technician know of our 'emergency'. Regrettably, she couldn't reach my partner, who was on a ranch call in Denton. But two other vets and their families showed up. If Dr. Vest couldn't be here, I'd hoped Fred would be the only other person with me during the surgery. More people around could mean more problems. In hindsight, though, having backup would have been a good idea.

Running over to me, Fred said, "Doc, I'll pull my truck 'round back—and we'll figure on how we're goin' to do this."

One of the kids yelled out from his dad's car, "Oh, boy, I'm going to pet the panther." This whole event made me nervous, so the boy's excitement didn't help. Always anticipating potential for trouble, Tracy came to the rescue, "Doc, why don't I sit on those kids, and just tell everyone else to wait out front." I relaxed a bit—knowing full well our gutsy technician would take care of everything, while still remaining two steps ahead of us.

Looking over the large solid crate in the back of Fred's truck, I shook my head. "Landsberry, what have you gotten me into this time?" My only sense of security came from viewing the numerous large screws bolting down the wooden slabs.

"I know this is kinda sudden, Doc," Fred explained. "But when my brother told me about the closing of that animal farm near his place in Yakima, I knew we had to move quickly. Barry said it was a small, private compound, and some of the older animals had already been euthanized by the time he heard about it. But he was able to save at least seven of them—a giraffe, two greyhounds, and four horses. His friends are taking care of 'em while he helps me out here for a few weeks."

When rumbling sounds came from inside the crate, Fred cajoled the cat. "Molly Brown, it's okay, we're here now…" Acting like a proud father, he fondly patted the crate's door, saying, "Doc, Molly's not tamed yet. She's just three years old and 110 pounds…so she's a baby." To Fred, every animal was a 'baby'.

I shouldn't have been surprised by Fred's casual attitude. Nothing ever fazed him. Seldom conforming to others' expectations, no one ever saw him in the customary horse trainer's attire, or even a western hat. On this particular evening, with Molly, he had shown up in cut-offs, flip-flop sandals, and a bright blue Hawaiian shirt.

Anxious to know what the cat looked like, I tried peeking through one of the many air holes in her container. Her deep growl made me jump back. The box was trembling…and Molly wanted out.

In the midst of planning the unloading strategy, Tracy read aloud from a letter attached to the crate. It was from Eric Mandel, Molly's former handler: *To whom it may concern. Molly Brown was raised in captivity, and kept in a pen. But I never handled her outside of the fencing. Although I was unable to spend a lot of time with her, I did brush her hair-coat and pat her head at feeding time. If trained, I think she can be friendly. Good luck. Eric.*

This didn't give us much to go on, other than he 'thinks' she can be friendly. We needed to proceed as cautiously as possible. Getting a tranquilizer to Molly without unscrewing the bolts was hopeless—and giving her an injection was out of the question. Even if I could reach her, I knew better than to administer a sedative to an agitated wild cat; it could kill her.

"Let's get 'er unloaded," I said. Molly shifted about when we lifted and carried the huge crate from the truck. Fred and I struggled to keep the crate moving and Molly's weight balanced at the same time. The back door to the clinic's hospital was too narrow. "Turn the box sideways," I yelled, "...and Tracy, get the cage door open and ready for her." A murderous roar came bellowing out from the box. Preventing Molly's escape was a priority right now. And I'd already decided if she got loose—our clinic was 'For Sale'.

Inside, with the box in position, Fred instructed, "We'll drop the side panel and let her walk into the cage." In an even voice, he smiled and continued, "When Molly steps out...you quickly move the carton away, and I'll close the cage door." There were a million and one flaws to this, but I didn't have a better idea. I had to trust that Fred knew what he was doing. The crate weighed as much as I did. But I'd manage—there was just no other way to do this.

"Ready?" asked Fred, "...ready?"

"Ready," I answered, as Fred began removing one bolt at a time. Now hissing, Molly hunkered down in the corner of the box. I held fast to the edge of the heavy paneling, crooning, "Whoa, now...kitty, kitty." That didn't do anything for her, but it made me feel better.

With the last bolt pulled, the slab door dislodged—crashing down against the bottom of the stainless steel cage. But Molly didn't walk out as planned. Hugging the corner of the box, she continued her hissing complaints. "Quick," I said, "Fred, use the broom handle to get her moving." As soon as he poked inside with the handle, there was a sharp, snapping crack.

"What happened?" I asked.

She broke it in half, " he said, "...so I think she's mad enough to come out now." Sure enough, Molly didn't just walk out of the crate—she lunged out at full speed.

Everything happened within a fraction of a second. I pulled the crate away—and Fred slammed the door and latch, saying, "We've got 'er!"

It was all a blur...and my adrenalin was pumping. "It worked!" I shouted.

"Good job, " Tracy gasped, with her last held-breath.

"Can we see the mountain lion now?" hollered a small boy from behind the closed kennel doors.

Freely moving about in her cage, Molly became extremely vocal. Sounding four times larger than any cat her size—her thunderous roars reverberated through the building. Folks still in the waiting room scattered. We heard one mother exclaim, as she scooped up her child and shot out the door, "It's getting late—we'll see the leopard at the zoo instead." Relieved, we couldn't help but laugh when thinking Molly had accomplished what we couldn't.

Fred and I sat on the kennel room floor, exhausted, knowing we still had the major work ahead of us. We sat there for a long time, just staring at Molly and marveling at her majestic beauty. He sighed...then, I sighed. She was a gorgeous beast, and even had a calming effect on us as she began pacing back and forth—showing enormous power in her stride. Her tawny brown body was long and muscular. In the clinic's bright light, her hazel eyes dilated...and gave her a kind look. Fred looked for his reflection in those large eyes—while I continued to ogle at the size of her forearms.

Molly's hisses began alternating with purrs, and she stopped her pacing to groom herself. When she licked her huge paws and spread her pads, the true length of her fangs and glistening claws were evidence of how lethal she could be.

Moving closer to her cage, Fred began soothing Molly in low humming-tones. Neither Tracy nor I uttered a peep as Fred seemed to mesmerize the cat with softly spoken words. Molly rolled over on her side. Well, I'll be damned, I thought. Reaching through the bars, Fred began slowly stroking the fur on Molly's back and neck. Wondering what strange magic he possessed, I whispered over to Tracy, "I can't believe what I'm seeing. How does he do that?"

Moving a little closer, I hoped she'd let me touch her, too. But her sudden, staccato grumbles set me straight.

Motioning us to back away, Fred lay on his side next to Molly's cage. Offering her a bite of canned cat food from the palm of his hand, which she gently took, he then held a small bowl of water between the metal bars. And Tracy and I watched in amazement as Molly contentedly lapped it up.

Within an hour, Fred had enticed the cougar to play. Propped on his elbow, he dangled an old piece of cotton rope in front of her, and Molly began batting at it as though she were a kitten playing with yarn. "Unbelievable," Tracy and I both murmured, as the cat purred. "She'll be ready for surgery by midnight," Fred said.

Making the necessary preparations, Tracy and I agreed that administering the necessary anesthetic would be challenging.

Molly might still have some reprisal at the moment the injected medicines begin to sting. And my assistant emphasized what I already knew, "Even a playful swipe could tear ya from stem to stern." We had just one chance to knock her out.

To fill the waiting time, Tracy decided to dash home and finish the dinner she'd started before we called her in. I wasn't relaxed enough to eat, but thought I'd grab some cold leftovers when I got home… not realizing I wouldn't make it home until breakfast. Fred, loving every minute of his new bond with Molly, took a snooze next to her cage so she'd become accustomed to his scent and constant presence.

At midnight, fetching two lariats and stretching a loop in each lasso, Fred slipped one hoop around Molly's neck, and I slid the other around the hock of her left rear leg. Keeping her calm, we waited—careful not to spook her. Then, with our feet firmly planted at the base of the latched door, on the count of three we jerked the slack from the ropes—with Fred snubbing Molly's head against the bars, as I secured her rump.

Molly had no time to react as Tracy plunged the needle of 'sleep juice' deep into her thigh muscle—exactly where it needed to go. Her hand withdrew from the velvet fur with an empty syringe, and she exhaled, "Whew…it's in!"

We waited, still holding Molly snug. "She's liable to explode," I said. We waited longer…but still no reaction. Molly hadn't flinched, and was still purring. "Tracy, are you sure you got it in?"

"I'm sure," she said, "…every single drop."

We shrugged our shoulders, as Fred said, "Let 'er go." With a tug on the end of the cord, we released our grip. Molly started to chomp down on the rope's loose end, then suddenly shook her head in a dizzy delight. Slowly slumping down, she rolled over and began snoring.

"Boy, that's quick-actin' stuff," Fred exclaimed, as Tracy quickly pulled up the gurney.

Lifting Molly into our arms, neither Fred nor I realized she'd be so heavy—or plump. Maneuvering her limp body onto the gurney, we wheeled it toward the surgical suite. When the ever-caring Fred noticed some extra fat swinging on the cat's belly, he said he was already planning a healthier diet for her.

Molly was in a sleep state—and Tracy began clipping the cat's hair in preparation for the operation. Stopping for a moment to admire the animal, my technician said, "I'm so jealous. Look at Molly's eyelashes, they're two inches long."

Beginning the incision for the ovarian hysterectomy, I couldn't help but talk to the cat. "Molly, this is for your own good. Without us, you wouldn't have had a home to go to."

The surgery proceeded well—only the cougar wasn't the usual ten-pound cat I was accustomed to. All her parts were of a grand scale.

The right ovary was tight, and removing it created the only real difficulty. I needed to tie off the trunk of the major blood vessels. But I'd seen water hoses smaller than her arteries and veins. Concerned about not causing undue hemorrhage, we proceeded with laborious attention to each and every stitch.

Molly's respirations and heartbeats remained rhythmic and steady. And we only needed to turn the knob of the anesthesia machine twice to increase the depth of her sleep. Looking at the clock as we moved forward into the de-clawing process, we knew each paw would take longer than it took for the entire reproductive alteration. Each of Molly's eighteen toes was a separate surgery within itself.

At this point, I was glad all three of us were working together so well. Tracy's arms fatigued when holding Molly's front legs, and Fred had to support the cat's rear paws while I stitched each digit's vascular supply and sutured the skin over the exposed knuckles.

Roll after roll of gauze and non-adhesive tape was used to cover her massive paws. I reckoned she'd chew the bandages off, but the best place to awaken from the anesthesia was back in Fred's wooden crate—since the decision had been made to let her recuperate at his farm.

The clock struck 3 A.M., and the surgery was complete. But we had one more task. Exchanging our sterile latex gloves for leather ones, Fred and I began the work of cranking the bolts back into the crate's heavy panels. With this done, we laid Molly on a soft stack of towels in the middle of the box, latching the panel door closed just as it was when she first arrived.

Every muscle of my body ached…and I could barely gather strength to help Fred lift and carry the shipping crate back to his truck again.

"Where are you going to keep her?" I asked.

Agreeing to call me daily with updates on Molly's healing, the trainer vigorously shook my hand—and winked. "Y'all come out and see."

All I could think of then was sleep. It was Saturday…and I was grateful for that. Now maybe I, too, could recuperate on Sunday.

* * * * *

Karen and I took Fred up on his invitation. After church service the following week, we drove to the outskirts of Celina. Curious to see how Molly was doing in her new surrounding, I also wanted to take time in removing her multiple bandages.

Greeting us in the same laid-back manner as his brother would, Barry told us we'd be in for a surprise when we saw Molly's 'hacienda', as he called it. At first, we thought he'd made a mistake when he headed toward a large, southwestern cottage. "Aren't you going in the wrong direction, Barry?" asked my wife.

"Not at all, this is *her* place," he said. At the massive entranceway, he swung open two custom-made, mahogany Spanish doors inlaid with scrolled ironwork and orange, stained-glass panels. Continuing across an expansive, tiled veranda that led directly into the open living area, Fred's whimsical side became evident. He'd given the entire place a jungle decor with bold greens and yellows. Hassocks and oversized rattan chairs were deep and inviting. Bright, floral-patterned pillows were everywhere, and tropical ceiling fans twirled overhead. Sliding glass doors opened to the outside patio, where two oblong pools were being fed from surrounding rock-ledged fountains. The view made Karen gasp. "Oh, this is beautiful—and a whole lot nicer than our house."

Fred had just come in from a swim and was lying next to Molly on the cool tiles. Barefoot, and still in his trunks, he motioned us over. "Come on in…Doc."

"You did *all* this for Molly?" I asked.

"No, this was an old guesthouse I had remodeled last year. But, as you can see, a lot of special additions have been made for Molly. Those swinging doors over there are easy for her to open by herself so she can get to her food bowls.

Molly didn't seem pleased by our intrusion—but too content and lazy to make a fuss—she just yawned, laid back and closed her eyes.

"Who took off all her bandages?" I asked.

Fred was as nonchalant as ever, "I did, Doc...I really didn't want to bother you more than I already had. And besides, I kinda looked forward to seeing the expression on your face when you saw how our baby was livin' now."

Karen couldn't resist. "Fred, this house is incredible. If I get de-clawed and spayed...can I come live here, too?" At that, she took off her shoes and, sitting on the floor next to Molly, began petting the drowsy feline. Molly stretched out when Karen massaged the downy fur on the big cat's stomach.

I thought for sure she'd now let me do the same. But as soon as I reached out my hand to touch her, her left eye popped open and a faint growl told me where I stood. Maybe she sensed I still had some trepidation.

I wondered if I'd ever develop her friendship. I also wondered why it was so important to me. After all, I'd worked with so many wild creatures, with no need to keep an ongoing connection with them. But there was something different about Molly. I couldn't put my finger on it. Perhaps I was saddened by the fact that she was one of the last of her species—an endangered breed. In a very few years, there may be none of her kind left.

I didn't see Molly again for several months. Fred had called me out to his place to treat one of his spotted mares for an abscessed hoof. I couldn't resist asking, "After all this time, Fred, do you think Molly will let me pet her now?"

"Sure, Doc…nowadays, she lets everyone pet her…she lo-oves people," Fred drawled with confidence.

I boldly walked into Molly's 'casa'—strolling over to her, talking in comforting tones. But I'll be…I didn't get but six feet from her when she let loose with one of her low, raspy hisses. As she started to move toward me, I instinctively backed up, turned, and took off. When I looked over my shoulder, she was just standing there—seemingly pleased with herself. If I didn't know better, I could swear she was testing me.

I never tried to get near her again, and will admit to feeling a little badly about it. But Fred, always empathetic, makes me feel better whenever he gives me news about his critters. He continues to thank me and tell me how well Molly is getting along. And he was especially delighted when several local teachers began taking their classes out to his farm for educational field trips.

I'd known about this, since my son was lucky enough to be a part of one excursion. K.C. said the students were always asking for return trips…and some had volunteered to help out at the farm on weekends. This came as no surprise. The gifted trainer's boundless enthusiasm, knowledge and profound respect for each animal was graciously shared through hands-on lessons and petting visits with the endangered ones, including everyone's favorite—Molly.

Blowing in the Wind

hickening black clouds appeared ominous. The last of the sun's orange streaks were fading across the parched, brown pastures as I cruised out past the McKemy ranch gate. Dreading the abrupt shifts of our Texas weather, and cursing the effects of our recent drought...I prayed we'd get a good, soaking drizzle.

Dusk ebbed, and boiling winds of red sand came rolling in from the west. A red-violet haze marked the horizon like a wall of fire. The sight gave me an uneasy, eerie feeling, and I sensed that something was terribly wrong. My partner's voice blasted from the speaker of the dashboard's two-way radio. "Doc! Unit #1...Call your uncle...Seven Star has been hit! Base, clear."

There it was...the terror I felt in my gut...TORNADO.

The knots in my stomach tightened as I screeched Ol' Blue to a stop at the nearest pay phone. Uncle Grump and Aunt Sadie's line was busy. I tried dialing the bunkhouse number...no answer.

Then the barn number…no answer. Attempting to keep myself calm, I even dialed the number for a neighboring ranch…no answer. "Com'on…com'on…somebody, please answer…"

I couldn't keep this up. I needed to get out there. Calling Tracy at Twin Oaks, I was brief. "Tracy, pack everything you can think that'll cover any situation…and be ready to roll when I get there. Have you heard anything from anyone at Seven Star?"

"Sadie called to say they're okay. But your uncle sounded pretty rattled. Try callin' him again."

On the second try, my uncle picked up the receiver at the family's ranch house. "Izzat you, sonny? Hello…hello?" With so much static on the line, I could barely hear. Over the bad connection, I could only make out a lot of noise and some of my uncle's shouts to his ranch hands. "Rex…try nailin' that tarp over yonder…and Sammy…hand me that bucket."

All I said was, "I'm on my way."

"Good…'cause it's bad…." He started to say more just as the phone went dead.

Ready and waiting when I honked the horn, Tracy hoisted boxes of medicines and bandages into the bed of the truck. We'd both seen the devastation from Texas twisters before. A few years earlier, in Joplin, Michael Cook's place had been peeled from the earth's surface and dropped into the Red River. He was Tracy's cousin. Fortunately, Michael, his wife, Jen, and Tracy's two young nieces survived by hiding in a grain silo just moments before the funnel cloud tore the walls of their home from the concrete foundation. We all pitched in to do whatever was needed. I spent three days helping him round up his steers. And Dr. Vest took a couple of days with Jen and the kids trying to salvage the family's belongings. We covered whatever was found with sheets of plastic. A year later, Michael built again—on the same spot.

I didn't know what, if anything, would still be standing at Seven Star. But I knew the only important thing—my folks had made it through.

I kept Ol' Blue's accelerator smashed to the floorboard. In the rearview mirror, reflections of fence posts flicked by as the broken, white highway line turned into one continuous ribbon. Heading toward Roaring Springs, a dry-hole town fifty miles east of Lubbock, Tracy asked how long it'd take for us to reach the ranch.

Watching the speedometer peg eighty and more, I remarked, "About three hours…at this pace." With no one else on the road, we stared straight ahead into the mind-numbing darkness.

Zooming past the rocky plateaus of Jacksboro, we raced across the flat plains near Seymour…then down into the bottom of the Palo Duro canyon to emerge near Guthrie—within sight of the sheer, multi-colored clay walls of Mother Earth's tabletop.

Suddenly hit with torrential rain, our view was obscured…and we slowed to a crawl. Becoming quiet, Tracy said little as we continued to drive at a snail's pace, being met with images we knew only too well. Not much of Roaring Springs was left. One farmhouse after another was totally destroyed…while at odd times, an undisturbed framed picture hung over a mantle…or a dog's food bowl would still be resting in its place on the owner's back porch. The church I attended as a kid was leveled, except for the cross and steeple-top.

Finally, Ol' Blue rumbled across the cattle guard marking the entrance to Seven Star Ranch. Able to catch only a glimpse of a flickering light in the distance, Tracy sounded frightened. "That's where we're goin'? Doc, that must be ten miles into the middle of nowhere."

"Actually, seven…" I began, before recognizing the first of many bizarre findings left in the tornado's wake. Focusing the headlights, we spotted a broken section of the large Seven Star sign…with the remainder nowhere in sight. "Geeze, look at that enormous, flat boulder of sandstone over yonder…it use'ta sit way up there," I said, as I moved the spotlight toward a far hill.

Slamming on the brakes, I jumped out of the cab at the sight of something very familiar. A big chunk of crumpled metal sat in the middle of a barren pasture…the remains of Uncle Grump's truck. Rolling down her window, Tracy yelled, "Doc, what is it?"

Wiping rain from my eyes, I tried to focus. I knew my uncle hadn't been in it, but the engine was still running and the dome light was on. Its windows were gone, and the radio had been sucked out. A splintered two-by-four had impaled itself through the driver's seat. The keys weren't in the ignition…and there were no bloodstains…but my uncle's sunglasses were lying unbroken on the console. The rear axle was bent, and all four tires were gone…along with the hood.

The sight left me speechless. We were six hard miles away from the main house. Walking past the beams of our headlamps over to Tracy, I tried to describe the truck's condition. But she shook her head in disbelief, "That's impossible—how can the motor be idling?"

Climbing back on board, I mumbled, "...don't have a clue. It looks like it rolled across the landscape like a tumbleweed. The roof is crushed, but there's not one dent on the fenders. It might've just dropped from the sky."

Soaked to the bone, I grabbed a towel to blot off my face and hands. There'd be no way I could think about dry clothes 'til we were at the ranch.

Shifting into 4-wheel drive, our tires kept skidding as we headed down the muddy road. Ol' Blue bucked and weaved ...while chunks of wet earth-clods continually slapped mud onto the windshield. "Whoa, lookie here..." Tracy exclaimed. From what we could tell, this might have been the spot where the tornado touched down. The flattened grove of trees was a dead giveaway. But we'd have to wait until daylight the next day before much of anything more could be seen.

A white-chested steer jumped and ran off when my spotlights illuminated his face, catching the reflection in his eyes. We stopped, in need of a breather before moving forward. That was when we became aware of a heavy, racy smell.

"Good gawd..." Tracy uttered. Seeing three bloated carcasses lying side-by-side, I then realized this was only the beginning. Grabbing my poncho, I told Tracy to remain in the truck. Holding my high-powered flashlight, I sloshed over toward the lifeless Watusi cows, and walking between the maimed bodies, managed to count at least eighteen.

Never one to sit in one place for long, Tracy pulled on her boots and tromped over to me. "Just look at this place." Shielding her eyes from the steady rain, she pointed toward a distant spot. "What's that weird thing over there...looks like the propellers of a plane." What once had been a towering windmill now lay flat, with its steel blades contorted ...jutting up from the earth like a misshapen anchor.

Despite the heavy weather, and overcome with curiosity, we searched around before heading back to Ol' Blue. As I picked up a branding iron from a ranch I knew to be twenty miles away, Tracy found a city light pole, and a leather saddle stuck in the briars. I recognized it as belonging to Sammy, my uncle's top ranch hand.

We came across more cows. Steam was rising from the still-warm bodies and damp hair-coats. At dawn, buzzards would be there to pick the bones clean of meat. "...poor critters," I mumbled to myself, walking up to a large bull curled in a ball with his ribs crushed and horns broken away from his skull. "He must've felt nothin'," I said. "Look at the frozen stare in his eyes."

"No...I'd rather not," Tracy whispered. "How much wind does it take to carry away cattle and trucks?"

My denim jeans were soaked to the stitches and splattered with mud. Water began seeping over the top of my boots, when I hollered, "Tracy, let's get out of here and back on down the road."

Lagging behind me, she began yelling at me through the downpour, "Wait...what's that noise? Do ya hear it...it's a calf!"

Baa...baa came faintly out from the dark. I spun around, searching, thinking the winds were playing tricks on us. But the cries were heard again. "Tracy, where is he...can ya see him?"

We both saw it at once...the silhouette of a dead long-horn cow about twenty feet from us. Making my way over to it and kneeling down, I saw something I didn't think possible.

Trying to escape from his dead mother's womb was a newborn. The muzzle, ears, and front hooves of a two-minute-old calf were emerging from the vulva of the dead cow.

Clutching what I could of the baby's slimy legs, I tried to fully expose its head, and shouted for Tracy, "Go get the O.B. chains from the truck…" *Baa…baa* insisted the calf.

"Hold on, 'lil fella," she yelled, "I'ma comin'."

At this point, mud and rain became the least of my concerns. Securing the dallies around the calf's forelegs, I used my right hand to guide the baby's head clear of the pelvic outlet. Straining and pulling, I needed to leverage myself by pushing my boots against the cow's rump. The calf's cries got stronger as his chest came through the pelvic canal. "Com'on, son…all we need now is your hindquarters."

After one more tug, Tracy cheered, "He's out!" With that, the calf slid up onto my chest.

Holding the baby by his hind legs, I lifted him up. A swift slap on his rear told us he was definitely alive. Too young to moo, he began crying nonstop…*baa…baa…baa.*

As I rushed for the truck with the orphan over my shoulders, Tracy excitedly exclaimed, "She's a heifer…and she'll need some nourishment as soon as possible." Then, remembering Sammy's saddle, she turned back just long enough to pick it up and carry it to the truck.

Despite the mud, Ol' Blue found traction in the road's worn ruts. And our worries subsided as soon as the stone house came into view. My spotlight gave us enough vision to see that parts of the roof were gone, and a portion of the rear kitchen wall had collapsed. But the rest of the family structure stood solid. Water was spewing from a broken main, and the corral appeared to be in shambles.

Standing and waiting on the porch with his propane lantern held high, my uncle waved…giving us a ready smile. "Lookie who's here, Mama."

Tracy felt she knew my Uncle Grump and Aunt Sadie since she talked to them so often on the phone, but she'd never been out to the ranch to meet them. Although few were close enough to call my uncle a friend, most ranchers found him likable. A hard man with a soft core, he spoke few words of endearment. On the other hand, everyone found my aunt a downright joy to be around. With her wonderful round face and dimpled cheeks, she always looked happy. She loved her own cooking, especially her thick, buttermilk pancakes…and over the years, became a mite chubby.

Uncle Grump again called out, "Mama…lookie who's here…"

The screen door flew open, and the additional draft set the winds to whistling through the shattered windows. My uncle's basset hound, General Jackson, came out to greet us, whimpering a little to let us know he'd suffered a cut on his tail from the flying glass. As I bent to console him, my aunt came at me with her arms open. "Y'all com'on in, ya hear?" Standing on the tips of her toes to hug my neck, she then playfully pushed me away. "Son…you're some sort of gamy to the smell…best you keep downwind…but it's sure good to see ya."

I didn't take offense…she didn't know what we'd been doing. My jeans were coated with mud, manure, and birthing fluids…and neither Tracy nor I noticed the odors. But Jackson's nose tweaked high in the air and he ambled away, turning his back on such a reeking smell.

Though acting as if nothing unusual had happened, I knew Uncle Grump was elated to see us. The leathery wrinkles on his face seemed to disappear as he thumbed his hat back. And he took to Tracy like she was his long lost daughter, wrapping his arms around her in a bear hug. During their greeting, I went to fetch the newborn.

Proudly holding the calf, I announced, "Tracy and I brought ya a new heifer from the north pasture."

"I ain't got no cows in the north pasture," my uncle frowned.

"Ya do now…eighteen or more dead cows, a mangled bull, and a whole lot of steers on the run." After explaining what had happened, I added, "We saw one steer with a 'question mark' blaze on its flank standing not far from a doe. But both of 'em jumped and ran."

Overhearing us as he came inside, after working on trying to plug the hole in the side of the kitchen, Sammy interrupted, "Grump…that's gotta be the same steer was pinned up in the southwest canyon by them hay bales. I sure wanna find 'im again."

"Naw…impossible," my uncle growled.

Suddenly everyone began talking at once, trying to explain the unexplainable. Still standing there with the calf in my arms, I looked down at her, knowing she needed tending to. "Are ya hungry?"

"Put the calf down here, sonny…" directed my aunt.

Stooping to lay the white-faced heifer on a thick, plaid blanket in front of the couch, the newborn squirmed and cried, as my Aunt Sadie took over. "Now, don't you fret, 'lil girl. I'm fixin' to care for ya…"

"Go git some goat's milk from the freezer, Sammy," my uncle ordered.

"Ya ain't got no freezer…nope, not no more," the Hispanic lad's voice dropped. Normally cheerful, he began sounding sullen and depressed, "…ain't got no bunkhouse…no tractor…no barn …no…"

Tracy stopped him from going on, "Hush up, Sammy …we know things will get better. Go out to Doc's truck and y'all will find a surprise…somethin' that belongs to you." Sammy's mouth dropped open, but he couldn't say anything. He just bolted out the door.

Laughing, sweet Aunt Sadie wanted everyone to see the bright side. "Ain't got no electricity, but I can make a baby bottle…and sonny brought us some birthin' milk… so we can feed this tiny critter." Following her sure instincts, she fashioned a milk feeder from a nipple and small coke bottle. Then, still in her rubber galoshes, she sat on the floor cross-legged, tucking her full, print skirt between her knees. Stroking the calf's long ears, she patiently taught the orphan how to nurse. As the heifer raised its head from her lap to begin sucking from the bottle, Aunt Sadie sighed, "…there, she's got it now."

At that moment, I again thanked my lucky stars for my technician. When I'd asked Tracy to prepare for any situation, she realized there'd be orphaned calves during this storm…so she added colostrum to our emergency supplies. Rich in antibodies, this 'first milk' was just what the newborn needed. And, at a time like this, it made no difference whether it was warm or cold.

"Now, y'all just dry your bones…and sit. And sonny, you go git out of them smelly clothes. Ain't no more we can do tonight."

Sammy came back in grinning and clutching the precious saddle, as Uncle Grump agreed. "Yep…we'll just hav'ta wait and pick up the rest of the pieces…com' mornin'."

Barn Cat's Dilemma

Jostling over littered acreage on the east side of my aunt and uncle's ranch, my trusty four-wheeled drive, Ol' Blue, closely followed Aunt Sadie in her borrowed jeep. Still surveying the extent of damage to the ranch and its livestock, we spotted three large, perfectly formed circles above the rise—each about a quarter-mile wide. Standing out in stark contrast to the rest of the landscape, looking like the crop-circles folks talk about, these were just formed by the fierce velocity of yesterday's tornado touching down at Seven Star.

Though part of this destructive path was seen last night, it was even more astonishing to now view the full impact of the storm's aftermath. Torn and uprooted cottonwood trees lined Glass Bottom Creek—stacked in rows like bales of harvested straw. Hundreds of tumbleweeds were still wildly drifting across the landscape. Woody vines of sumac shrubs had been whirled into tight knots. And, while broken twigs of wild holly were scattered all about, their berries, surprisingly, remained attached. Skeletal remnants of the thorny mesquites were eerie looking— their rough, hardwood bark having been literally stripped off by the force of winds.

Ahead of us, two pumping oil wells appeared intact. The hammerhead rigs were still moaning, swirling, and grinding. And their rhythmic sounds were hypnotic. *Thump...swish...thud... thump...swish.* Only a small leak and a broken cable were apparent. But the worn painted letters bearing the company's original name, West Seven Oil, had been sandblasted away by the twister. *Thud...thump...swish.*

While none of the wells spit more than a bucket a day anymore, the sharp odor of fumes still lingered. Uncle Grump turned his nose up. "Whew, and...hey, get rid of that," he said as he grabbed the cigarette perpetually hanging from Sammy's lips. Having worked with my uncle for years, Sammy was the one hand who should have known better. Smashing the glowing filter-tip on Ol' Blue's floorboard, my uncle hopped out of the cab and rushed over to the large, red shut-off valve. "This damn thing's not movin'," he grunted. The oil field was really a relic of times past, and the valve wheel was rusty and corroded. "Sammy, come gimme a hand." The slick-haired young bronc rider from New Mexico was all muscle. And between the two of them, the old wheel valve finally creaked and moved enough to be shut off.

When Aunt Sadie and Tracy pulled up next to the oldest of the ancient wooden derricks, Tracy said she was shocked to see it still standing—and wondered how and why. It was beyond me, too. According to my dad, Uncle Grump had been threatening to tear it down since before I was born, although I'm sure nostalgia kept him from taking such dramatic action. Oddly enough, even the tornado didn't help him out.

In its day, West Seven's 'Big Dipper' was one of the deepest wells known—with the tallest towering lattice-derrick in the county. Built in the early 1930s, there wasn't another that could compare to it. For years, a seemingly unlimited number of barrels were produced, until the last few drops of crude were spilled on to the red sands. Uncle Grump became wistful whenever he laid eyes on the rustic structure.

But a few years back, while attempting some repairs, Sammy had survived a bad fall through the rotting timbers, and wide scars were still noticeable on his left arm. Both men stood there in front of the teetering historical site, deep in reverie: one remembering jubilation and joyous fiddle sounds on party nights when any of the wells 'came in'; the other, too young to have experienced those times, thinking, instead, of the awful day when his arm was caught and broken in three places.

We continued driving slowly through the twisted debris of household goods and furniture haphazardly strewn across the vast acreage. Sammy pointed off to a clump on our right resembling a scrap field. "Gawd, there's the tractor wheels, and there's the hood from Grump's truck that Doc and Tracy saw last night…six miles from here."

I spotted one of the toilets from the bunkhouse, when my uncle exclaimed, "Hey, those are my good pants in that tree. OH, NO…lookie there…Sadie's baby grand piano!"

Lots of folks in other parts have no understanding of the trail of ruin caused by these twisters. It was even hard for me to understand. And I was always moved by how folks here stoically endure and rebuild after each of Mother Nature's fits. There's an abiding belief that "Ya play with the hand you're dealt…" my uncle would say.

Aunt Sadie, as much at home on barren prairie as any cowboy, held her arms out toward the canyon walls, where cattle were huddled below. Turning Ol' Blue onto a wagon trail leading down past the mouth of the jagged rocks, we got a better view of the small herd from a ledge…the same ledge where the piano now sat. My uncle anxiously began counting, "Six… twelve…forty-two…eighty…Yep, there's damn ner' a hundred and four, as I count 'em. That's good…they're all here. Sure wish I coulda said the same about my longhorns in the south pasture."

Tracy and I trekked over to where Aunt Sadie's piano was lying. At first, it looked as if it had been picked up and set down without so much as a scratch. But when we got up to it, we saw that all the ivory keys were gone, plucked out like white teeth. The polished woods that Aunt Sadie so lovingly buffed and dusted for fifty years were splintered beyond repair, and the fine-tuned strings and brass fittings were gutted.

A long-eared jackrabbit darted out from behind a prickly pear, as Uncle Grump came rushing to catch up with us. Looking out toward the ranch, he said we were two miles from their living room. All of these these things from their home had been carried that far by the winds.

"Lookie here," I said, lifting the lid on the three-legged piano bench found nearby. "There's still sheet music inside the seat. Let's see, there's 'Rose Marie', 'This Ol' House', and 'Blowing in the Wind'." I swallowed, "Geeze…isn't that a spooky coincidence?"

"Ain't it?" Uncle Grump dropped to his knees, swearing, "Damn this country…a man works all his life, and sixty years are lost in sixty seconds." Then, staggering to his feet with a burst of anger I'd never seen from him, he grabbed under the piano's keyboard with both hands and forcibly shoved the hollow box of sound over the cliff. It cracked and shattered on the rocks below. And I was glad Aunt Sadie wasn't there to see it. Up to this point, I'd been wondering just how long he'd be able to stay calm. Never one to show his feelings, Uncle Grump was a man who kept his emotions buried deeper than the oil. But for that brief moment, he looked like a Texas Ranger with six-guns blasting away. Suddenly, straightening his bandana and snubbing the brim of his hat, he pulled himself together, saying, "There… what's done is done." Dusting off his knees and looking down on the cattle, he ordered, "Let's go see if any of 'em are hurt."

Aunt Sadie became withdrawn and silent. And we later discovered why. During the time we thought she was waiting at the jeep, she'd also been hiking around and gathering other belongings entwined in the roots of the sage. She saw her piano toppling over the cliff. Her oven and refrigerator were also found crumpled like paper against the boulders. She never said a word…but we knew it was the piano she'd be thinking about— and missing. Then and there, I began planning for some way we could all pitch in and get her another one.

One tiny surprise helped her perk up and smile again. "Look what I found," she yelled over to us. Holding it up, high in the air for everyone to see, was her discovery of a single, unbroken, fresh hen's egg. Stopping to talk about the strangeness of this find, we heard a loud MEOW echoing throughout the canyon.

"That's Mouseketeer!" Uncle Grump hollered, and called to his old barn cat, "Here, kitty…kitty."

There was an answering MEOW…but we couldn't tell where it was coming from. "He must be down in the arroyo," my aunt said…but he'll come up, now that he knows we're here."

"Yeah, he will," my uncle agreed. "Let's go see after them cows right now, and then we'll come back and git 'im." Grabbing my medicine bag, I made my way down the steep embankment, with Uncle Grump and Sammy two steps behind me. Other than being spooked and uneasy, the herd appeared to be in pretty good shape. We only needed to rope two steers to stitch a few minor lacerations. Slowly easing our way through the rest of the cattle, we checked on each cow, calf and steer to find—with great relief—that none were injured or lame.

After climbing back up to the top of the ledge, and hearing the cat's cry again, we puzzled over where he could be when Tracy pointed towards the sky. "There!" she said.

Craning our necks back, we all looked up to see Mouseketeer on the edge of the old derrick's platform. "Ohmigod…" Uncle Grump said, "he's going to jump."

"No…no…" I said, "…he'll climb down."

"You've got to go git 'im," he insisted.

"Are you talking to me? He's *your* cat." Turning to Tracy, I mumbled under my breath, "Can you believe this? My uncle wants me to shinny up the side of that ancient ruin to rescue his scraggly ol' barn cat."

Shading his eyes with the brim of his hat, Uncle Grump said, "It's your damn fault he's up ther'…'cause he hates veterinarians…and that's why he run'd up ther'."

"He either ran up there scared of the tornado, or the tornado dropped him there. Either way, it has nothin' to do with me," I said.

Obviously funning with me, his voice changed. And with a hoarse laugh, he looked me square in the eyes, saying, "Then he won't mind ya fetchin' 'im down."

Debating with my uncle would be even crazier than going up the derrick—and I'd never been able to say 'no' to him. "Oka…ay, oka…ay," I moaned reluctantly.

Sammy quickly handed me his chaps, lariat, and leather gloves. And Aunt Sadie gave me one of the pillowcases she'd found among the scattered goods. "Be careful," she warned, "…and don't you dare fall."

I began to awkwardly scale the squeaking lumbers of the rickety old tower—wondering to myself why Sammy wasn't doing this. Though I knew everyone expected the vet to do the humane thing…even if it meant risking his life. Trying to stay calm, I took one rung of the frail ladder at a time—slowly stretching for the next step and the next.

Forty feet up, feeling one of the boards begin to crack beneath my soles, I held on tightly to what I could. "You can do it," Uncle Grump hollered up at me, "…just don't look down." Inching my way up, I continued climbing.

Reaching the crow's nest at the top, where the derrick slightly swayed, I began crooning to Mouseketeer, "Here…sweet kitty." In spite of his circumstances, this ol' cat wasn't glad to see me. Hissing and growling, he scampered to the other side of the platform plank…still frightened. Crawling on my hands and knees toward him, while feeling for the pillowcase tucked under my belt, I was ready to make my move. But he stood his ground, and the gray hair on his back bristled. He was kind of cute, I thought…with his stubby whiskers as short as his bobbed tail. Eyeball to eyeball we stared, as he dug his sharp claws into the decaying wood. "Don't hurt 'im," Aunt Sadie shouted from below.

Feeling like a matador looking down the nostrils of a bull, my only worry was that *I'd* be the one getting hurt. One false move and maybe the derrick would crumble beneath us—or Mouseketeer would leap off. A brief, sudden gust of wind came up and the steeple shifted again. "Oh, hell…" I groaned, as my sweaty palms stuck to the splintered wood surface like suction cups. Scooting a little closer, thinking it best to talk to the cat like my uncle would, I commanded, "Gitcher' butt in the sack…and iffin' you jump, I'll kill ya!" Mouseketeer's eyes blinked and, unbelievably, he began purring. Stunned, I grabbed open the pillowcase, and he walked right inside. Closing the protective sack before he could change his mind, I hollered down, "I've got 'im."

"Don't drop my cat!" Uncle Grump yelled.

After tying the sack to my belt to free my hands, I started the long climb down. Sammy and my uncle cheered and hooted on every step of my descent. As we carefully eased downward— one crossbar at a time—Mouseketeer managed to embed his claws in the leather covering the side of my thigh, and I doubted chaps were ever designed for this purpose.

Again, the boards beneath my boots began to bow and creak…and I instinctively reached over my head for some type of anchoring. As a few planks began pulling away from the derrick's main frame, I thought, "… I'm goin' to die here!"

"Jump to the center-post of the well…use it like a fireman's pole," yelled Sammy. With no time to consider options, and the final foothold pulling away…I dove for the metal drilling shaft and, holding on for dear life, went slip-sliding all the way to the ground.

With heavy dust billowing out at the moment of my hard landing, the kinfolk came running. "Are you okay?" they asked in unison. As I shakily stood up, my uncle immediately reached for the sack secured to my belt and untied it. Mousketeer's head popped out of the pillowcase, and Uncle Grump grabbed him and hugged him. "My baby!" Rubbing his own cheek next to the cat's face—the two ol' timers cuddled, whiskers against whiskers. "We've got some birthin' milk at the house, little fella," my uncle soothed.

"Don'tcha mean those bottles of colostrum Tracy brought in for your orphaned calves?" I corrected.

Paying no attention to me, my uncle went on and on with promises to his cat. "Next time a twister comes, you're comin' down in the cellar with us. And when we rebuild the barn, I'm goin' to build a special cathouse, just for you." He stroked the barn cat's dusty fur, holding him tighter than he would a lost child. This uncharacteristic display of affection caught us all by surprise.

As I limped toward the jeep, Sammy asked, "Hey, Doc… would ya mind fetchin' my rope from atop the derrick? Ya left it up there." Looking up, I could see the end of his lariat dangling from the broken boards of the oil well's platform.

Through clenched teeth, I said, "Wait 'til the next tornado blows it off."

"Go up yonder and get it yourself," Tracy urged, playfully poking him in the ribs.

A devilish grin spread across the cowhand's face as he chuckled. "Only a dern fool would climb up there...sorry, Doc."

When the Time Has Come

rowing up on the ranch, it wasn't unusual to hear
an often-repeated line from my dad. "If you've got
livestock...then, one day, you're going to have dead-
stock." For a long time, I tried to protect my son
from this reality—which may have been a mistake. Lately, I'd had
some concern that he didn't have any idea about the downside
of my profession.

During the summer vacation before entering fifth grade,
he'd meet me at the clinic for lunch almost every day. This was
good, old-fashioned 'father and son' time...and I always looked
forward to it.

On one such day, Elijah Pardee had just called—and the
father of two was crying unashamedly. "Doc, he's down..." Trying
to gain control of his emotions, he simply said, "...it's the end
of the road for my guy."

His horse, Scrapper, had been battling bone cancer for a long time. We both knew what had to be done, so my response was immediate. "I'll be right there, Eli,"

At that precise moment, my devilish son bounded through the clinic door ready for lunch. I told him we needed to put it off, because one of my longtime animal patients was dying…and he needed me.

"Why can't I go with you?" asked K.C.

Wishing to spare him, I strongly suggested he stay at the clinic with Tracy and Dr. Vest, "…'cause I gotta put Scrapper to sleep."

Jumping down from his perched position on a stool, K.C. suddenly seemed mature. "That's too bad…but I'm goin', too. You might need my help."

Hesitating, I said, "Son…this may be hard. Are you sure you want to come?"

Obviously, his mind was set. Tucking in his shirttail and grabbing his cowboy hat, he shadowed me out the door. "Yep, I'ma comin', Dad. *Then,* can we go to lunch?"

His comment made me doubt he fully understood the gravity of the situation. He wasn't taking 'no' for an answer, and I was impressed with his eagerness to help. But, at the same time, the Pardee family was grieving…and I knew this was going to be a traumatic experience for them.

Arriving at Eli's farm, I found exactly what I feared. Their Quarter horse was lying on his side, unable to stand any longer. A backhoe-tractor was nearby, and a deep grave had been prepared not far from the debilitated animal. The tearful family of five had on their best clothes. Eli's daughter Sarah, a girl of nine years, was wearing her favorite green jeans, and her brother John, five or six, wore his fringed chaps. After hugging both their mother, Ginny, and their Grandma Helen, the loving family gathered in a circle around Scrapper, holding hands. They'd just had their own personal service, expressing gratitude for Scrapper's life and offering peace—as they would for a dying relative.

Not wanting to interrupt this moment for them, I waited near the truck until Eli motioned me over. None of the family members wanted this day to come, but they didn't want their beloved pet to live in pain.

Being firm with my son, I said, "Now, you stay put right here...don't you move...this is a time of privacy for these folks." Then, taking my medicine bag containing the euthanasia solution, I went over to the family's side.

Their bay companion had lived five years beyond what had been expected. When a diagnosis was first made, the pathologist estimated he'd last only six months. True to his name, Scrapper lived on against the odds. But the malignant carcinoma eventually metastasized to his lungs, liver and kidneys.

As I knelt by the horse's head, gently stroking his mane... Scrapper's eyes seemed to reflect his acceptance. He, too, knew it was time. A nudge from his muzzle and a soft groan told me he was tired of fighting his condition. When I looked over to Eli and nodded, the family closed their eyes and tightly clasped their hands together as I slipped the lethal injection into Scrapper's vein. He didn't move. Faithfully administering the fatal dose, and standing up, I quietly announced, "...he's no longer with us." It was a somber moment.

Eli stepped away from his family and said simply, "Thank ya, Doc." Grandma Helen smiled at me to show her appreciation. The others were still trying to cope with the finality of the loss. Turning, I saw that my son was sitting on the tailgate of Ol' Blue and watching everything. And I wondered how this affected him. Everyone agreed it had been for the best...but what would K.C. think of me. And was he aware of what had just taken place? Then, standing on the back end of the truck, he yelled out at the top of his lungs, "Hey, Dad...IS HE DEAD YET?"

The suddenness of the question was too much for Sarah, who buried her head into her grandma's neck and sobbed. Embarrassment reddened my face, but K.C. wasn't finished. "I'M HONGREE...let's go eat, Dad."

K.C.'s cold intrusion made things worse for everyone. Even me...for I'd treated Scrapper since he was a foal...and felt an undeniable bond with him. At that moment, I wanted to become invisible...but there was no place to hide.

What could I say? I stood frozen...rooted on the spot. But Grandma suddenly saved me when her stomach began to grumble...loudly and repeatedly. "Ohmilord," she chuckled..."Pardon me." Sarah and her mom, even Eli, giggled a little under their breaths. Unexpectedly, Eli wiped the tears from his cheeks...and laughed. It was the relief they all needed. Grandma Helen's blush resembled mine, and she again had to reluctantly apologize, "Excuse me..."

Rushing toward the truck, I hoped to quiet my son before any more outbursts. He sensed my displeasure, but I didn't think it right to scold him. I told myself he was just being a kid. But, again, he voiced his plea, "Can we pu-leeze go to lunch, now… can we?"

Putting my finger to my lips, I motioned for him to hush up. Did he still not understand? I couldn't believe Karen and I had raised such a rude boy, who thought only of himself. I needed to explain there was a time and place to speak one's mind. So I began, "Son…right now, nothing should be said…and maybe we should go."

Climbing into the cab, and closing the door…K.C. looked over at me. "Dad, it's a good thing they called ya to stop the horse's sufferin'." I needed to hear this. Maybe he hadn't meant to be disrespectful after all.

"K.C., it might also have been a good thing if Eli and his family knew you felt that way. If you remember, almost every summer Scrapper used to let you and Sarah ride him around the pasture. He's one of the reasons why you know how to ride so well today."

Without saying another word, he opened the door, hopped out of the cab…and, removing his hat, walked over to Scrapper. On his knees, he leaned over and said something in the horse's ear, while patting him on the neck. Then getting up and grabbing Eli's hand, he said, "Mr. Pardee, I'm real sorry ya lost your friend…he was the best horse I ever knew."

Before my very eyes…my son was finally growing up.

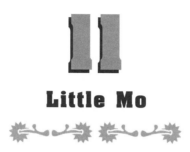

Little Mo

I stopped short...alarmed by the strange silence. I'd just opened the back door to the clinic, but didn't hear a single bark. It had been a frigid night, so I told myself the animals were still sleeping. Then a muffled noise came from the treatment area—someone was sobbing. This was definitely an odd beginning to the morning. Walking toward the sound, I began to guardedly check all the rooms along the corridor separating the hospital wards.

Then I saw her...hovering over a small cardboard box on the exam table. "Rachel?" Our receptionist quickly wiped her eyes, trying to regain her composure when she saw me. Giving her a quick hug, I had to ask, "...what's wrong?"

"...this...I found it on our doorstep when I came in. I'm so glad you're here early, Doc...'cause I sure can't bring myself to open it."

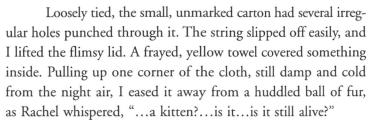

Loosely tied, the small, unmarked carton had several irregular holes punched through it. The string slipped off easily, and I lifted the flimsy lid. A frayed, yellow towel covered something inside. Pulling up one corner of the cloth, still damp and cold from the night air, I eased it away from a huddled ball of fur, as Rachel whispered, "…a kitten?…is it…is it still alive?"

Carefully cupping the small creature in my hands, I felt for a heartbeat. The chest of the abandoned infant moved in and out, but her eyes weren't open yet, and the length of her body wasn't as long as my thumb. Her nose was pink, and her ears were pink. "Yea…she's alive…but chilled, hungry, and barely a part of this world. She can't weigh more than two ounces…and must be only about three or four days old."

The tiny calico looked like a fuzzy caterpillar. But at the feel of warmth…her mouth opened and she squeaked. Walking in at that moment, Tracy and Dr. Vest were surprised to see Rachel pacing back and forth, swearing at whoever was so uncaring as to leave a baby kitten out alone in sub-zero weather.

No one said another word. We'd been down this road before. Always in sync with one another, we each moved quickly to do what was necessary. Tracy fetched a warm towel from the dryer, and I began massaging vitality into the little life. Dr. Vest reached for the incubator and hooked oxygen lines to the glass womb, while Tracy rigged a tube-feeding apparatus to provide nourishment from baby formula.

The unwanted kitty didn't struggle at all. After administering a few cc's of formula, Tracy placed her in our life-support box. And we continued watching her vital signs to see how, or if, she would respond.

Lashing out again at the irresponsible person who did this, Rachel was having trouble coping with both her anger and sadness when Tracy interrupted, "There really are jerks out there… but they must'a thought they were doin' the right thing by leavin' the box at a vet's hospital."

We weren't sure if the calico would make it. But, for the moment, she was sleeping soundly. Almost simultaneously, my partner and I said, "We'll need to feed her every two hours. Just let her rest right now…and keep the oxygen flowing and…"

"I've got her, doctors…" confirmed Tracy. And we knew nothing more needed to be said. When it came to raising orphans, our technician had an amazing track record.

Taking a moment to talk about the realities before us, my partner asked, "What are we gonna do now?…ya know we can't adopt every stray animal left here."

I had to agree. "I know…I know…but I don't guess there's a right or a wrong answer here. Every case is different…we'll just take it a moment at a time and see how things unfold."

The kitten was much too small to survive on her own. Vets everywhere face this type of decision almost daily. There were only two choices: 'go for broke' with ongoing treatments…or euthanasia. The 'logical' business decision supported the later. Still….

Rachel's high-pitched shout prevented us from thinking further. "Docs…y'all com' here."

As we approached the incubator, Tracy and Rachel were smiling. Lying on her back, the kitten was using her back legs to support a doll-bottle that Tracy had prepared. Clutching the nipple between her front paws, the infant began sucking. It was quite a maneuver for one so young, but she managed—on her own—to contentedly nurse down the formula.

"We named her Mo…," said Rachel,"…'cause every time the teeny bottle runs empty, she wants mor'."

No one could deny their motherly instincts…nor would we want to. Tracy and Rachel were delighted with the kitten's positive response—it turned the day around for all of us.

My partner and I looked at one another…knowing the decision was made. That evening, I carried Mo home in the pocket of my smock…giving her the required formula throughout the night. Dr. Vest did the same on the following night. We'd bring her into the clinic during the day, and Tracy and Rachel took turns feeding her and wiping her bottom with cotton balls. Rich and I continued to alternate the caregiver role…even awakening most nights to Mo's faint cries when she was ready for her bottle. The routine was no different than if she'd been a newborn child.

It didn't take but a few days for the calico to progress from sleeping in a shoebox on my nightstand to the softness of my pillow…and me. An occasional nip on my earlobe was apparently the security she needed. When her eyes finally opened, Rich and I laughed at the thought that we were certainly the largest, ugliest 'mother cats' she could have had.

Mo's adoring nature captured our hearts, and a month passed in no time. Mostly white, with black and yellow splotches, the kitten's beauty was beginning to show. A thin, gold stripe down her nose matched her funny personality. When her eyes sparkled with excitement and mischief, she'd go bounding through the clinic like she owned the place. She did. Her appetite shifted from formula to baby food…and that was fine. But she resisted moving on, preferring chicken and rice baby food to anything else. With four people doting on her every desire, she was spoiled…of course. When Tracy finally coaxed her to move on to solid, adult cat food, we knew the time had come to find her a permanent home. It needed to be done, sooner or later.

Only one name immediately popped into my head… Sarah Pardee. Her close-knit family had just lost their horse, Scrapper. I knew from experience how much they loved animals, and how well they treated their sweet little dachshund, Bart. Even though Mo had no fear of dogs, I still wasn't sure if the two of them would get along.

I reluctantly put the kitten in a carrier along with her toys and drove out to the farm, telling myself that even though the Pardee family may not have a lot of money, they would be the perfect family. Oddly, I felt like some sort of social worker, about to approach unwary folks with a solicitation. "Please…will you adopt…?"

Sarah hadn't come home from school when I arrived. So this was my chance to chat with Eli and Ginny, and tell them about the plan. When I broached the subject of gifting their daughter with a newly orphaned animal, they were both pleased and moved. But after some hesitation, they confessed that animal-care bills were a constant crunch in their budget…and they already felt stretched to the limit.

Assuring the couple they'd be doing this for us, I told them to consider our clinic a 'sponsor' for Mo. We would provide immunizations, spaying and any other medical treatments whenever needed. The soft-voiced Ginny then said, "Well…it won't do any harm to at least take a look at this kitten of yours…"

One look was all it took…they were sold. Mo was up to her usual, charming tricks and won them over with her loud staccato-purring and outlandish stretching positions.

I finally spotted Sarah and her brother, John, down the road, coming home together. When John ran into the barn to milk the cow as part of his after-school chores, Sarah came over to talk with us. At first, she thought her mom was cuddling a cat belonging to a neighbor…and Ginny didn't let on. But as her mother leaned over asking Sarah to hold the kitten for a while, Mo eyed the young girl's long, light-brown braids and began wildly batting at them. Sarah was totally enchanted…enveloping the irresistible kitten in her arms and hugging her tightly.

The delight on his daughter's face gave Eli the confidence to tell her, "Doc, 'ere…wonders if you'd like ta have this 'lil cat. She was abandoned…and they've all been takin' care of her 'til she was old enough to go to a nice home. They thought of you… what d'ya think, girl?"

The look in Sarah's eyes as she glanced over at me was beyond any description…more than justifying our efforts, sleepless nights, and early decision to raise Mo.

I left the farm feeling better, though somewhat heavyhearted, knowing I'd miss that crazy calico. But Sarah was happy, and Mo would be happy with her. That's all that mattered.

When we did have another chance to see the two of them, Mo again added something special to our day. This time, looking as wide as she was tall, she strutted through the clinic like it was still hers…and that afternoon gave birth to her first and only litter at the clinic. There wasn't a single calico in the bunch, but the four healthy newborns—each squeaking to be fed on demand—were all white.

As soon as Sarah brought home the new brood, the dog was right there at Mo's side. He watched over her babies, and even helped to groom them until they were weaned. The kittens proved to be chips off the 'ol block, and as nutty as Mo ever was. Since everyone wanted a cat "...just like Mo," Sarah had no trouble placing them with eager new owners.

Becoming inseparable pals, Sarah, Mo and Bart greeted me enthusiastically whenever I visited the farm to treat Eli's livestock. On my last trip, with Mo boisterously rubbing against my leg, I bent down to pet her...then looked up to thank the caring girl. "Ya done real good, Sarah. I wish we could save all the critters left at our door."

To this day, Mo's chart is the only one still permanently marked: *Free of Charge.*

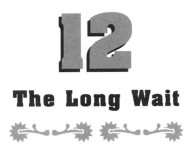

The Long Wait

r. Rich Vest combed his fingers through the cotton-like fur of the American Eskimo dog. Talking softly to the injured pup as though he could be understood, he gently rubbed Puff's ear and murmured, "You're gonna be fine, boy." At this, the young pooch smacked his lips and trustingly rested his head on my partner's forearm.

We gingerly carried the fluffy white dog into the radiology room, laying him on the X-ray table to position his right side against the film cassette in order to snap several pictures. The sweet-natured animal fixed his large brown eyes on mine as I patted his outer thigh, but he appeared to have no physical sensation. "We're gonna find out what's wrong with your back, Puff," I said, as I wiped a small puddle of dribbled urine away from his hair-coat. Then after carefully wrapping the dog in a thick towel—holding him in a way that wouldn't allow movement to his spine—Dr. Vest slowly moved him to his cage.

Since we were now running late with scheduled appointments, I began checking in on our other patients. On this particular day, each case had a familiar and common situation: owners who waited until the last minute before getting help for their companions.

There was the feisty tan cocker with bushy whiskers who, for six days, had severe diarrhea from eating pork bones; then there was the orange, long-haired alley-cat who suffered for weeks from a scratched cornea—unable to open his irritated, swollen eyelid from the ulceration; and then, the gray tabby who got her tail caught in the garage door, injuring it more than ten days before she was brought to the clinic. Luckily, it wasn't broken. But I couldn't help wondering, as I often did: Why do they wait? Why don't they bring them in sooner? It's not that they don't care—they do. We saw this again and again—even when Mary Bean almost ran out of time for her three-year-old sidekick, Puff.

An attractive olive-skinned woman in her fifties, Mary Bean limped a bit from slight arthritis, and it made her seem older than her years. With her gray-brown hair tied tightly in a bun, and her characteristic horn-rimmed glasses, she looked every inch the vision of a stereotypical librarian. She was, without a doubt, the last person in the world you'd figure to be a private investigator—and probably the reason she was so good at it. She'd often brag about her intriguing life. "Me and Puff used to work with the FBI. And I've used my psychic abilities, inherited from my mother and grandmother, to help the Dallas police in solving a couple of dozen crimes." I remembered seeing occasional articles about Mary in the local paper.

Perhaps it was the stress of her line of work, sleep deprivation, or the adrenaline-high that comes with intense adventure—but Dr. Vest and I agreed that this lady often seemed confused, and, as they say, didn't seem to be 'playing with a full deck'. Her first calls about Puff had thrown me.

"Doc, he won't drink any water. He's limping on his front leg, and he acts like he might bite me when I touch his side. What do you think? I gave him two aspirin about ten minutes ago."

It was hot enough outside to pop corn on the stalk, so I couldn't figure why Puff wasn't interested in water. I asked her how long the lameness and behavior change had been going on, and if Puff was still able to eat.

"Let's see, it all started last Thursday," she said. "And, yeah, he ate."

"How bad is the limp?"

"Not bad. There's no swelling or cuts…and his pads are cool. Oh, Doc, it's probably just a sprain. I'll give the aspirin more time to work."

"Can you bring him to the clinic?"

"No, I'm sure he'll be okay." Since the abrupt dial tone meant our conversation was over, I ended up muttering to myself that I hoped she'd bring him in if he didn't improve. That was Tuesday morning. Mary didn't call back until Friday afternoon; and this time she sounded distressed. "Doc, Puff still hasn't been drinking any water…he's going to dehydrate. He's not walking on his back legs, and he pooped in his sleep."

"Whoa, Mary, whoa…let's back up a step." I interrupted. "Did you say back legs? I thought he was limping slightly on one front paw."

"Doctor, you're not listening," she snapped impatiently. "He won't drink...does he need fluids? I gave him two more aspirin. His front leg is fine. But, now, he's draggin' his back legs around the house." Casually, she added, "I wonder if he got hit by a car?"

"Why would you think that?"

"Because Puff has a big tire mark on his side," she added.

"Tire mark?" I nearly choked on the coffee I'd been sipping. "Tire mark?"

I leaned my forehead against the wall—aghast—and Rich took the receiver from my hand in time to hear Mary's explanation. "Puff and I were on a serious stakeout. I was involved in some note taking. But at one point, I noticed him lyin' against the curb, actin' kinda weak. Let's see, that was over a week ago...and he's still not drinking any water."

Dr. Vest interrupted, "Mrs. Bean, you get that dog into this clinic...and now!"

We waited anxiously—running out of what little patience we had left. Then, finally, on Saturday morning, Mary came through the door pulling Puff behind her as he tugged on the end of his leash. His eyes looked alert, and his forequarters moved just fine. Though all his vital signs appeared normal, Puff's hindquarters were fallen...and he had no control of his bladder or bowel functions. Using his front legs to move, he valiantly dragged his back legs across the tile floor. And there—on his side—was a large, black oil spot bearing the unmistakable imprint of tread lines. Mary chattered nonstop during Dr. Vest's neurological exam, saying Puff was still not drinking. But water intake was the least of her pet's problems.

We suspected the worst, but didn't have the final diagnosis until we studied the developed Xrays. Pointing to the film, I said, "Mary, Puff has a broken back. The bony spinal column has shifted, causing trauma to the spinal cord. Permanent nerve damage is a real possibility. But, for now, he still has some pain reflex."

"That's the good news," said Dr. Vest. "The bad news is he could still be paralyzed after the surgery—and never walk again."

"We're going to try to stabilize the fracture," I added, feeling it necessary to repeat, "…but if little Puff makes one wrong move, the spinal cord can be forever damaged."

I wasn't sure she took this in, because she still seemed overly obsessed with water. "Can he have a drink of water?" Mary asked again, as Tracy fetched a bowl and Puff freely lapped it up.

"He'll get plenty of fluids during his lengthy surgery," my partner assured her.

"Can I please take him home tomorrow?" urged Mary.

"We'll call you when we're done," Dr. Vest and I said simultaneously.

Puff's surgery was upgraded to critical. Clinically speaking, bones may be bones. But, emotionally, nothing compares to the kind of overwhelming pressure a doctor feels when operating on the spinal cord. Two stainless steel plates were placed alongside the spine to align the vertebral column. Fractured bony fragments were delicately wired into position while medications to reduce infection soaked the tissues surrounding the central nervous system. Puff's strong back muscles were tightly secured —fixed into a rigid posture for as long as it would take for the necessary fusion to occur.

Some three hours later, I called Mary as promised. "Only time will tell now. The motility in his hindquarters should gradually return. *But if*…and this is a big *but if*…if he's still paralyzed at the end of six days or more, then we'll worry."

Fortunately, Puff beat the odds and came through surgery with all the positive signs for a full recovery. After a week of steady recuperation in the clinic, it was time for Mary to take him home. As usual, the nervous psychic lady asked, "Did he drink any water?" Not waiting for an answer or wanting to hear what else I might suggest, she quickly said, "Then, he'll be okay."

"Yes, ma'am. But I need to see him at least once a week. We've got a long road ahead of us, and I want to remove those skin sutures in about two weeks."

Puff's tail wagged slowly as Mary caressed him, "Don't you fret, my little buddy, the stars are in your favor—and I'll get you a fresh bowl of water when we get home."

I believed Mary understood our concerns and instructions. So we were surprised when she didn't return any of our calls. Dr. Vest and I left message after message on her answering machine. And we'd regularly ask one another if there'd been any word from her.

Three months later, Tracy waltzed into our office with a frolicking white pooch at her heels. "Docs, can you guess who this is?"

His tongue was flapping. His tail was wagging. And that telltale black spot on his side had faded to a dull gray. "Lemme see," I said, as Mary stopped in the doorway. "Could this be Puff?" I ran my hands down the canine's back and felt each suture still in place. "Mary, I thought I told you…I needed to see him every week."

"Well," she hedged. "Sorry, but I've been workin' on an assignment for the CIA in San Antonio. But Puff's been drinkin' plenty of water. Besides…my readin' of the Tarot cards said he'd be just fine."

Rich shook his head in amazement, and said, "Mary, did you know we thought he was dead?"

"Oh, no," she laughed. "If that had happened, I'da called ya for a refund."

Tracy couldn't help but cuddle Puff, while I sat on the floor with him and finally began removing his sutures. He licked my hand and rolled on his back while I scratched his belly. A stream of urine sprayed like a fountain into the air. "Welp, that works."

"I told ya, all along…" said Mary, "…all he needed was a drink of water."

Mary appeared jubilant, and kindly offered us her special metaphysical services as her way of showing gratitude. "Docs, maybe I can read your palms?"

We chimed in together, "No, ma'am, but thanks anyway."

As our eccentric client happily strolled out of the office with Puff jumping and barking at her side, my partner whispered, "Frankly, Doc…I think there's a crack in Mary's crystal ball."

Ferrets, Frogs 'n Fishes

 didn't dare look up, or Rachel would be pointing to another exam room. This time, our authoritative receptionist snagged Dr. Vest. "Go to Exam Room Two...and be careful, it's Julia Cope."

Too curious not to interrupt, I had to ask, "Don't tell me, did she bring in a gorilla with tattoos this time?"

"Nope, she's got a ferret in a pillowcase. But I'm warnin' Dr. Vest to be careful of *her,* not the ferret...'cause he doesn't know Julia yet."

An attractive young blond, Julia worked as a bartender at the local boot-scootin' tavern. On occasion, we'd treat the lame barrel horse she kept boarded at A.J. Hall's stable near the clinic.

"Shush, you two, I wanna hear what's goin' on in there," whispered Tracy, pretending to press her ear against the door of the room Julia had entered with the pillowcase in her arms. It wasn't necessary to listen in, though. Julia's husky voice was loud enough for everyone in the waiting room to hear.

"Dr. Vest, I'm still tryin' to tame Blackie. So he needs all his shots in case he gets loose…and his nails need trimmin', too. But maybe ya heard how I am 'bout the sight of needles…so if ya don't mind, I'll wait out front 'til you're done." At that, Julia rushed past us to the reception room.

For the next five minutes or so, each of us went about our business. After treating a client's white Persian for a slight ear infection, I wondered why there'd been no sign of my partner or the ferret. And Julia was still out front reading a magazine.

Suddenly, Rich's laughter pealed out from the room. I assumed he'd just untied the pillowcase, and got a look at the little ferret for the first time. More and more of these unusual animals were being domesticated. Distant relatives to the weasel, they're known as fast, persistent little hunters. But, with people, they could be either friendly or not…depending on how well they were tamed.

The suspense was killing me. "Maybe he needs your help, Tracy…take a peek."

With the door slightly open, we could see the examination table and my partner's back. The table looked like a lingerie counter at Macy's, with slips, bras and nighties spilling all around. Continuing to pull more of Julia's unmentionables from the case, Dr. Vest impatiently mumbled, "Where in the heck is that dern weasel?"

Then Blackie's tail slid out from beneath a pile of crumpled bed sheets. Laughing, I pushed open the door, "What's the matter in here?"

Rich jumped back in embarrassment and began shoving Julia's lingerie back into the case. We both grabbed for the slick-haired ferret, but true to his species, he squirmed away and hid inside the clothes bundle again. Frustrated, Tracy called Julia in to help.

"What's wrong?" the pretty girl asked, as she stood bare-foot in the doorway…a fetching sight in short shorts and an over-sized sweatshirt.

Holding up a pink nightgown, Dr. Vest lamely joked, "Julia…I don't think this needs a shot."

Blushing, Julia buried her face in her hands and apologized. Then deftly reaching into her laundry, she pulled out her frightened black ferret, petting and calming him.

We agreed she needed to stay with us during her pet's treatment. So while Tracy kept her busy chatting, my partner and I completed the necessary tasks as fast as possible, then let Blackie slip back into his hideout before he could take a nip at our fingers.

Tracy and Julia were good friends, and gabbed away like a couple of ducks in a box. Our technician had always been fascinated by Julia's many strategically placed tattoos…so she couldn't help but notice the new flag art on her ankle. Julia, anxious to show off, pulled Tracy over to the corner of the room, and with her back to us, whispered, "Oh…and I've got some other new ones ya gotta see." With that, she raised her shirt up over her head, "Well, Tracy…what do ya think?"

Normally my partner and I tuned out their conversations, but this time we looked up…wondering what all the secrecy was about. Mighty proud of the artwork, Julia turned around. "Doctors, you've seen everything else I own today…so, what the heck…why not my tattoos." To our complete surprise, she again pulled up her shirt to expose all.

"Ohmigod," gasped Dr. Vest. He was trying to keep his composure, but the sight of two colorful butterflies tattooed on Julia's bare breasts left him stunned. Lowering his eyes and quickly changing the subject, he handed Blackie over to Julia, assuring her that the young ferret should do well once he got a little older and more familiar with his new home.

Rachel came in to drag me away, letting me know I had another client waiting. So I left Julia, the ferret, and the butterflies…while complaining that my partner always had all the fun.

* * * * *

At first glance, I didn't see a soul in the next exam room and thought whoever was waiting had left. Then a small voice behind the table got my attention, "Mister…hey, mister?"

The door was open, and Rachel announced, "Doc, that young man, Freddy, needs your assistance." Peering around the large exam table, I looked down to see the pint-sized boy.

"Why, howdy, sir…How may I help you?"

"Mister…it's my frog, ya see…"

"Frog?…and what's the matter with your frog?" I asked, bending down to have a one-on-one discussion with the lad.

Reaching deep inside the front of his shirt, he pulled out a mottled-green street frog. "Here, it's his foot…see?" he said, shoving the creature into my face. "Can ya fix 'im?…my friend run'd over his foot with his bicycle. His toes be real hurt…SEE?"

Carefully taking the frog from his hands, I uttered a dramatic sigh. "Uh, huh!…this looks very serious, Freddy…we'll have to take him to our special treatment area." Standing at the door, Rachel winked at me and guided the four-year-old down the hall.

Circular lamps, machines, wires, and monitors helped to capture the boy's imagination. Rachel then gave him a glass of juice and let him sit in a large metal chair next to the table. Gaining confidence as he watched me, Freddy asked, "Are ya gonna use all this stuff on my frog?"

"If need be," I said, while noticing how smashed the frog's right rear leg actually was. His lateral claws were missing, and the metatarsal bones had been crushed. The vital interdigital webs were also severed. It's been said that some amphibians have the ability to regenerate wounded limbs. Though I'd never seen proof, I believed it to be true.

"…eh…I ain't got much money, mister."

"Yeah, well…we'll work somethin' out."

Freddy was quiet and serious while I took time deciding on the best course of action for his frog. Tape would be too heavy, and gauze would only get wet. After measuring the length of the frog's leg, I split a plastic soda straw, and then rigged a tiny splint. It would be strong enough to stabilize the fracture site, yet light enough for the frog to have use of its limb.

No one ever watched me as intently as that young man did. After soaking the frog's tissues with antibiotics, I placed his pet back into Freddy's waiting hands. And he gingerly put it inside a small box with air holes that Rachel had prepared.

"How much do I owe ya?" the little guy asked…while reaching in his pants pocket and retrieving six pennies.

"Have ya got a penny?" I asked.

"Yeah…I got six."

"Well, one oughta cover it."

Taking Freddy by the hand, I escorted him out front to his waiting mother, adding, "And you be sure to let me know how he does, okay?"

Holding the covered box tightly to his chest, Freddy strolled out of the office jabbering to his frog. Telling his mom all about the serious operation, he blurted out, "…and it was cheap, too."

* * * * *

Rinsing and drying my hands, I asked, "Who's next, Rachel?"

Handing me a phone message, she said, "It's Ella Raymond at the Josey Elementary School. You need to call her back."

While dialing, I wondered what kind of problem the popular second-grade teacher could be having.

Coming on the line, Mrs. Raymond asked, "Doc, I've got three sick classroom pets here…can you come out to the school?" Figuring the animals were too large for her to get them to the clinic, I asked about the nature of their illnesses.

"Our gerbil seems to be constipated, and the turtle has lost his energy. Even the goldfish won't eat. My students are very upset."

Convinced, momentarily, that someone on my staff had put her up to this, I politely told her that perhaps it would be practical, and cheaper, to replace the three animals with healthy ones rather than pay for a house call.

"Oh, no…no…that's not possible…the kids would know the difference," she emphatically replied. Since Ella had been one of my son's favorite teachers when he attended grade school, I felt a tinge of obligation to comply with her request and agreed to examine the ailing beasts at the school.

Twenty minutes later, my official clinic became the reading circle table of the second grade's classroom. The students had already gone home for the day when I began my examinations, assisted by the sweet-faced veteran teacher.

Herman's fuzzy rear was matted with feces and cage shavings. So while he wiggled, I gave him a good 'butt washing' under the sink, and showed Ella how to do the same. The gerbil's buckteeth chattered as he once again spun around, pain-free, on his exercise wheel.

It was immediately evident that Flash had turtle scurvy, a serious deficiency, and needed a vitamin shot plus a better diet. But administering shots to these tiny, soft-shelled creatures was always tricky. So, remembering a technique from medical school, I tickled her until she extended her leg, then quickly gave her the injection.

The teacher's sheepish grins were understandable. But her third case was a mind-bender. Holding the goldfish up to the light, I could see he'd swallowed a blue pebble from the bottom of his aquarium.

After telling Mrs. Raymond I wasn't sure how to get the rock out of Goldie's stomach…her next question caught me by surprise. "Can't you remove it surgically?"

Looking into her blue eyes for a long moment, trying to keep a straight face, I said, "With all due respect, surgery is not an option. The last fish I operated on ended up in a frying pan."

Ella giggled with embarrassment, saying she realized her question was absurd, but wondered if anything could be done for such a miniature fish. Goldie was just three inches long and an inch wide.

Holding the mini-size fish by his tail, I tried to shake the pebble loose. It didn't work. While filling a syringe with water, I teased Ella, "Can you drown a goldfish?...we'll know soon enough." I then attempted to flush the rock out...but, again, no luck.

Finally, in desperation, I gently squeezed Goldie's mid-section until her lips puckered, enabling me to see the tiny stone. Then, luckily, after inserting delicate forceps down her throat, I was able to grasp the stone and quickly retract it. For a split second, I wondered what my former medical instructors would have said to me if they could have seen me now.

Goldie, fully recovered, swam around in her bowl searching for food and ready to delight tomorrow's class. Ella Raymond agreed to change Flash's diet to ensure a longer life for the turtle. And, as for Herman...she said his young caregivers would be taught proper grooming procedures so the little critter could remain comfortable and energetic.

Ella was elated...and only then did I realize why she was such a good teacher. She went to extreme, sometimes impossible, lengths for her students. And I doubted if many others would care enough to do the same.

While driving back to the clinic, I laughed to myself... imagining how easy the days would be if all my patients were like today's—small enough to fit into the palm of my hand. But I never had a day like that again.

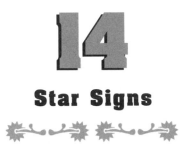

Star Signs

The windows were rolled down. In the hot, breezy air, Tracy's long ponytail bobbed from one shoulder to the other. Crossing over the iron bridge next to Sid Syler's hog farm, we were on our way to make one quick farm call before heading back to the hospital for more interviews with veterinary interns.

Our appointment book had only one of Rachel's distinctive scrawls: *This won't take long—cut three boar piglets*—meaning Sid wanted his pigs castrated. I aimed Ol' Blue across the cattle guard and slid to a stop, as Tracy jumped out to pop open the hatch to the vet-box.

"Wait, there's no one around…and Sid said he'd be waiting." We spotted a note tacked on the farrowing shed just as Rachel's voice blared out of the two-way radio, "Unit One. B.T. and ewe problem. Ag Barn…911."

Jumping into her seat, Tracy answered, "Base...we're rolling...Clear," and we took off again. Unfolding Sid's message, she read, *Doc—Sorry I missed you. Signs ain't right. Stars are in their bellies. Maybe next week.*

"What in the blazes does he mean by that?" she asked.

"Some call it folklore, but it's one of those beliefs Sid has. And, heaven forbid I might cross them."

"Cross what? What are ya talking about?"

"The stars...astrology. The signs, what they tell the rancher. Sid reads his *Farmers Almanac* every mornin'. He might plant his crops at midnight, in the rain, or during the Sign of the Twins to get a double-yield. And when he says, 'the stars are in the pig's belly', then I don't do any kind of surgery, because it means the blood supply is pooled in the abdomen. So, if you castrate, they'll bleed more. "

Tracy seemed dumbfounded. "I can't believe someone would practice such old thinking in this day and age."

I told her we'd get her a paperback on astrology so she could get a handle on it. "It has somethin' to do with gravity and the tides, the moon, stars and sun. And who knows what else. Sid's beliefs are common in these parts. What's more, he told me when the stars align with the signs in the pig's feet, then they won't bleed at all."

"Aw, Doc...you believe that?" was her next question. And I hoped it would be her last, since I didn't know much about the subject either.

"Don'tcha see, Tracy, Sid believes it, and that's what counts. And besides, if Sid said the signs were wrong, and one of those pigs bled to death after my operation…then I'd be the laughin' stock of the whole farmin' community."

Shaking her head in amazement, Tracy insisted on having the last word. "Look, this is Judge Sid Syler we're talkin' about—he's the damn judge for the Dallas County Court of Appeals. His decisions are gospel, so I'da thought he'd know better."

I wasn't going to argue about this. Driving past the lands of the Comancheria Trial, we both became silent…and my mind wandered. Tracy stared out the window. This was a place of reverie—the dry river basin beyond the Indian burial grounds. Arrowheads could still be found here. And it was easy to imagine thousands of Comanche teepees and their campfires lining the banks of what was once a wide, roaring river.

Turning right on the six-lane expressway, then left on Sandy Lake Road, Ol' Blue's dual rear wheels spun as the frame lifted over the railroad tracks. We bucked and rattled over the ruts leading down to the high school's agriculture barn and pulled up at the red metal lamb-shed.

It always bothered me to come here. In the ten years B.T.'s been the Ag instructor, he's yet to fix the gates to his ewe barn. Barney Travis knew less about lambing than our receptionist did. The man shouldn't be teaching, I thought. There's no telling what he'd gotten himself into this time. But I swore I wouldn't get involved in a long, drawn-out procedure—which usually happens whenever he calls.

Originally from New York, Barney was a 'transplant' and he spoke pretty good Texan, until he got excited. "Doc, I 'cawed' you guys as soon as I found the problem with Sharon Welch's lamb."

The worried young girl stood nervously waiting at the pen door. "How long has she been this way, Sharon?" I asked. Jiggling the latch open, I stooped down into the deep, bedding straw next to the Suffock ewe lying on her side, panting. She was trying to endure the pains of pregnancy labor. Tracy knelt by the wooly sheep's head, and I separated the matted fleece beneath her nubby tail. Her flank hair was stained with sweat, urine, and afterbirth fluids. "What tha hell…"

Stroking the lamb's black ears and patting the curly fuzz on her neck, Tracy suddenly glared up at Barney. "Omigod! She's…"

Sharon quickly said, "Doc, Mr. Travis said she was aborting her kid, and he put those things in her last night."

"Last night? And he told us he called as soon as he found the problem." My face turned red…and I was about to explode.

Tracy tried to calm my rising anger. "Doc…Doc…"

The two-year-old ewe's legs became rigid. Her trembling and straining made me focus on her condition, instead of Barney. I took a deep breath trying to bring down my racing pulse.

All the inept Barney could say was, "Her name is Bella."

After another torturous uterine contraction from the ewe, I tried to gather my wits and asked, "Did you do this?"

Barney had misinterpreted the symptoms of natural birth. Miscalculating a ewe's normal gestation period, as well as mis-diagnosing her premature delivery…he'd sutured the lips of the mother's vulva closed with a shoestring. Fashioning the plastic tip of the shoelace into a needle, he had blocked the newborn baby's escape from Bella's womb with a manmade zipper.

"Geeze, well did ya?" Mumbling a little, his eyes couldn't meet mine. In a feverish effort to keep Bella from going into shock, I reached for the scissors and grabbed an intravenous catheter.

A faint sound was heard as the kid's tongue tried to dart between the threaded lattice. I snipped one knot, then another. With each forceful contraction by Bella, small cuts on the baby's muzzle oozed red where the resisting laces had sliced the tender skin. As the laces were removed, the baby could finally breathe without struggling. One nostril flared, then the other. She bawled weakly. The rest of the kid's brow looked like it had been smashed against a window. I slipped a finger between her pressing skull and snipped the last of the woven threads. Her head and forefeet emerged.

With the kid safely in the pelvic outlet, I inserted an intravenous catheter into Bella's jugular vein as Tracy held her head. Reaching to assist the delivery, she monitored the IV drip, while my right hand guided the ears and neck, then shoulders. My left hand gripped both forelegs as one and pulled. Bella pushed, and I tugged… until the newborn popped from the canal into my arms. Exhaling in exhaustion, Bella greeted her baby with a weak *baaa*… and her kid answered *baaa…baaa*. Tracy and I couldn't help but smile as the two called back and forth to one another. There was something sweet and comforting about that sound.

Cleaning the mucus from the newborn's airway, thinking the abnormal delivery was done, Bella began to strain again.

"Doc," Tracy said, "Bella's still pushin'."

Sharon gasped, "She's having another contraction…twins!"

Reaching deep into the new mother's uterine body, I touched a breech fetus entangled in a web of swollen tissue. My fingers went numb as ten minutes of maneuvering went by, then twenty. Sweat was rolling down my back. And Bella just couldn't push any longer.

"Can you turn 'er?" Tracy suggested.

"I can't reach far enough. Bella's too small, and the unborn is packed like a sardine."

"What can we do?" asked Sharon. "Bella will die if we can't do something...Doc?" The thirteen-year-old had been struggling to hold back her tears.

How, I wondered, did a brief farm call for baby pigs turn into such a disaster? "Damn..." I grumbled under my breath, and faced Barney. "Bella's got to have a C-section right now. Any questions?"

Barney didn't dare open his mouth. He and I both knew Sharon couldn't afford such surgery. Bella's value was sentimental, and the risks were high—given her weak condition. But she was Sharon's pet. Barney nodded his consent to go ahead—he'd cover the costs.

Scooping Bella into my arms as Tracy capped the catheter, we rushed out. Barney and Sharon followed, with the freed newborn clutched against the girl's chest. Nothing was said until I opened the door of B.T.'s gray sedan. "But what about the mess?" he complained, as I laid the ewe gently on the rear seat of his family's car.

"What mess?" Tracy will stay with you to get the fluids goin' again for Bella. I laid the newborn on a small blanket on the front floorboard close to the warmth of the heater vent. "Barney, follow me to the clinic."

"And, Sharon, you ride with me." Picking up the mike, I called in to Rachel, "Unit one to base, we're comin' in *hot*... Clear."

"I'll rearrange appointments and have the surgery room ready. Clear," Rachel answered.

While pulling away, in my rearview mirror I could see what was happening in the sedan behind me. Tracy was mopping a pool of urine from Bella's behind, and Barney was fanning his face to avoid the pungent odors of new birth. I had to laugh at the sight.

Rushing through our hospital lobby, sheep pellets and blood droplets trailed behind us, marking our path down the hall and into the illuminated surgery room where Dr. Vest was waiting.

We moved the anesthetized ewe onto the stainless steel table. Bella's vital signs kept faltering. She'd been through the worst kind of punishment.

"She's in rough shape," my partner commented. "And, Doc, this fella standing here is our new intern, Steve Malone. I took the liberty of goin' through the formalities since you couldn't be here."

Tracy interrupted, "Docs, Bella's respiration and pulse are as stable as they're gonna get."

Making one long incision through the ewe's abdominal muscles, I briefly acknowledged Steve. "Welcome to our Texas-style practice...we're now proceeding with a C-section in an effort to save this mother ewe."

Bella's second offspring swiftly emerged from the confines of the left uterine horn. She voiced her freedom by bellowing. Just in time, I thought, as I began sewing at a frantic pace in order to minimize any more trauma. Dr. Vest clamped a bleeder, while Tracy snipped the suture material after I tied each knot. The ewe's skin was closed over the layers of stitched muscles before we placed her in recovery along with her healthy twins.

Peeling one bloody glove away, then the other—it looked like Dr. Vest was waiting on me to say more to Steve. "It's nice to meetcha, Dr. Malone. You'll be ridin' with Dr. Vest this afternoon…and you're fixin' to meet one of our favorite clients, Pete Channel, over at the Samuel Ranch."

Going out to the waiting room, I gave Sharon a wink, letting her know Bella and her babies were alive, and told her they'd stay with us for a few days of healing time. At the news, she hugged Rachel, Tracy, me—and even Barney. I'd never seen a girl so happy.

We realized Barney was trying to get things right when he attempted to apologize. "Doc, I promise I'll never diagnose another medical condition. And I'll bring you guys a check for the surgery and the hospital stay first thing in the morning."

I was beginning to think there just might be something to this astrology stuff. After all, Bella had twins during Gemini, the sign of the twins. I'd remember to tell Sid about this…he'd appreciate it.

At day's end, with time to finally go over Steve's résumé, I wondered if his stars aligned with ours. A day with Pete Channel on a Texas ranch would tell us a lot. Stars or no stars, we'd know then if this intern had what it takes. Dr. Vest and I had agreed we'd never hire an associate unless the signs were right—and only our clients and patients would let us know when that happened.

I didn't have to remain concerned about Barney, either. His conscience must have gotten the best of him. When he announced his early retirement the following week, the news came as a great relief to a lot of folks...especially me. Now, hopefully, future agriculture students would have a real chance to learn something about basic common sense when taking on respon-sibility for animals they care about. I was so pleased about the turn of events, I even accepted the high school's earlier offer to be an occasional guest lecturer for these eager students—many of whom could quite possibly become the future vets of Texas.

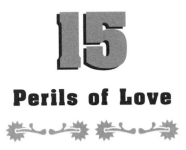

Perils of Love

repping for another routine day at the clinic, I groggily stood in front of the mirror, shaving. Catching sight of the emergency beeper still clipped to the elastic band of my underwear, I had to admit to myself that no day was ever 'routine'.

Sprawled at my feet was our ol' dog, Lugar, who took up this position every morning in his patient wait for morning rituals...when I poured my first cup of coffee and gave him his first biscuit treat of the day.

As if I hadn't noticed his presence, the 120-pound rottweiler loudly grunted and stretched. "Yeah, Lugar...I see ya," I said, patting him on the head as he rolled over on his back. "You've got a tough life, don'tcha fella? I wish all I had to do was eat and hold down the floor tiles."

Lugar grunted again when I stroked his smooth, black coat. After all, he'd been under stress lately. Several weeks ago, he needed to lift his head out of the food bowl long enough to breed with Mandy, his new mate. And, even then, he didn't do much work.

I finished dressing before going into the kitchen…and Lugar lumbered along behind. He was noisily crunching on his biscuit when K.C. came rushing in to hand me the cell phone. "Dad, here, it's some crazy lady." His sixth-grade classmates called everything and everybody 'crazy'. And Karen and I were hoping they'd soon grow out of this stage.

The 'crazy' lady was actually Jenny Harrison. She and her husband, Mike, were our new neighbors. The young couple from California had just bought the old stone house across the street. Mandy was their gorgeous, silky rottweiler. They adored this pooch and treated her as though she were an only child.

Lugar's ears perked and his nubby tail moved a little as I answered the distraught caller with, "Mandy did what? Take her …and it…to the clinic, Jenny. I'll be there shortly." He either recognized the names, or he spotted a second biscuit cupped in my hand. Whatever the reason, he barked when I told Karen that, according to Jenny, Mandy just aborted a puppy.

Hurriedly, I took off for our Twin Oaks Clinic, trying to remember the sequence of events leading up to Jenny's news.

* * * * *

Only a week after they moved in, the Harrisons asked if we'd consider arranging a match between our two dogs. They'd been impressed with everything about our Lugar, including his size and temperament. Their own pup was also in excellent condition, and even certified 'free' of hip dysplasia—the genetic pelvic arthritis every owner worries about.

She was the finest dog Lugar had ever laid eyes on. Though Mandy wasn't quite ready to breed, Lugar still acted as if she was a goddess. The two of them played and cavorted around our yard until exhaustion captured their senses. "She's flagging but not ready to stand," I told Mike.

Since their first date was a mating fiasco, Jenny brought Mandy by again a few days later. And Karen called to fill me in with the progress of their relationship. Apparently, Lugar wanted to skip any prolonged foreplay, but Mandy insisted on formalities. "It's just cat and mouse right now," Karen laughed, "...he's too heavy, and her rear end collapses whenever he tries to get near." I was confident they'd figure it out, but Karen was still concerned. "Well, he's gonna have a stroke first," she explained, "...his tongue's hanging longer than a jackrabbit's ears."

While emphasizing that no one has ever seen a dog die from breeding, Jenny piped in from the background, "You haven't seen him...that poor fella's been working three hours on a twenty-minute job."

We figured it would be a good idea to separate them until I got home. So when Mike and I arrived at my house at about the same time, the two of us actually tried to guide Mandy and Lugar into position, while Jenny and Karen coached from the sidelines.

Ultimately, we had to admit defeat, agreeing the only way to create this match was through artificial insemination.

Intent on following through, Mike arranged an appointment at the clinic. And though I'd done this procedure for other clients, my own dog was never involved before. Lugar never liked coming in to the hospital. But with Karen fussing over him and giving him an extra biscuit that day—all went according to plan. Barring any unusual complications, the signs were good that Mandy would finally have a chance at becoming pregnant.

* * * * *

When O' Blue rolled to a stop at the clinic, I kept thinking that Mandy couldn't possibly be aborting yet, since she was only two or three weeks into her sixty-one-day pregnancy. Barking and prancing when she saw me enter the kennel, she sure didn't act sick. While I took some time to examine the 'lil mother-to-be, Tracy asked, "What's the deal? Mrs. Harrison just dropped her off, and said you knew she was comin'."

"Jenny called me at home this morning…crying," I explained. "She said Mandy aborted a puppy on the living room floor. I told her to bring her and the pup into the clinic as soon as possible."

Interrupting, Tracy said, "She left a shoebox up front."

"What's in it?"

"Don't know…didn't want to look…I left the box alone for your inspection," she grimaced.

"Welp, Mandy's perfectly fine, and still as pregnant as she can be."

I went into the treatment area and lifted the lid off the shoebox. It appeared to contain nothing but a whole roll of crumpled paper towels. Layer by layer, I unfolded the coverings to see what was hidden beneath. It seemed strange that the paper was dry. Tracy couldn't help but peek over my shoulder. At first, we

saw something resembling a small head with eyes. Then I noticed
what looked like a dried umbilical cord extending from the tiny
body. The round torso was covered with mucus, but it was firm
to the touch and hard to identify.

As I rinsed it off at the sink, Tracy sighed, expecting to
see a dead puppy.

"Well, I'll be dang…No!" I laughed. "The cord is metal
and the body is plastic. It's a dead…ornament!"

"A what?….a what?" she repeated.

"An ornament—like the kind you hang on a Christmas
tree. It's chewed up…but it looks like a chubby bear. See? Here's
the head and eyes. And here on the bear's backside is a gold-foil
sticker saying *Made in Hong Kong*. Mandy must have coughed
it up during the night."

When Jenny got my call, she was still upset. "Doc, how
bad is it?"

"First off, Mandy's still healthy and very pregnant. And
secondly…this isn't a puppy."

"But I saw its eyes and its body," she argued.

"I assure you…this ain't no puppy, Jenny. Did you see the
sticker on the rear of the bear ornament with the printing *Made
in Hong Kong?*"

"Ornament? An ornament? Are you sure?"

"Let me put it this way, Jenny…out of the last two-
hundred litters I've delivered, I've never seen a pup born with a
gold sticker on its butt."

Jenny giggled with relief, but said, "Oh, Doc, I still think
you've got to be joking."

She knew it was no joke when, a little over five weeks later, their sweet rottweiler gave birth to eleven healthy puppies. Only two had Mandy's sleek looks, while the rest took after our husky ol' Lugar. But a family of rambunctious pups can terrorize a household.

Surprisingly, the Harrisons were letting the puppies have the run of their entire home. I probably should have warned them. But I knew they enjoyed 'spoiling' the brood and didn't want them confined to a single room or to a puppy-pen. So their little vandals toppled vases and chewed up the sofa and area rugs. It was only after they left scarring bite-marks on the corners of the couple's prized, antique armoire that Jenny and Mike announced, "…eight weeks of this…enough is enough." They adored the lovable puppies, but were happy and relieved to find a great home for each one. Reluctantly, they came to a decision. There would be no more 'created' love matches for Mandy.

Lugar put up with the boisterous pups gnawing and yanking on his sensitive ears for only a few days, as well. Then he, too, was done in. Cranky and overly tired to meet the demands of fatherhood, our good ol' boy contentedly returned to his lazy ways…revving up just enough daily excitement to satisfy his biscuit addiction.

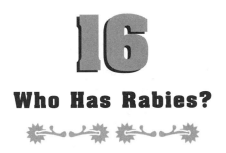

Who Has Rabies?

In the distance, a dust cloud barreled toward us, getting larger and larger. All the dogs on the ranch began howling at once. We were out on the mesa, in the middle of nowhere, doing sonogram procedures for each of Jake Gordan's mares. But at the approach of the speeding truck, with its red lights flashing an emergency, we stopped immediately.

"That's Hallie's truck," said Jake. "She's not only the cook and owner of Hallie's Café at the Fence Post Junction, but the mayor and sheriff, too."

I'd known the indomitable, red-haired Hallie since I was a kid. Her café was the only gathering spot in this remote valley. As her tires skidded to a stop in the sand, the ranch owner shouted, "Hallie, what's so important that ya hav'ta come way out here?"

The tough eighty-three-year-old didn't even get out of her truck. Looking directly over at me, she was blunt. "Doc, you gotta call your clinic right away. Rich Vest said somethin' 'bout rabies."

Jake quickly said, "Doc, go use the wall phone in the live-stock barn. It's the closest."

Racing past the lower pasture and up to the barn, I got Dr. Vest on the line after the first ring. "Rich, who has rabies?"

This was every vet's nightmare, and I prayed it was a false alarm. I'd been exposed five years earlier and had to endure the painful series of vaccine injections…a procedure I never wanted to go through again.

There was silence at the other end of the line. "Rich…can you hear me, are you still there?"

"Yea, Doc…do you remember Ranger, the German shep-herd puppy we saw on the Friday before you left? He was the little black 'n tan shepherd mix with multiple puncture wounds on his neck, face, and front legs."

"…the puppy from the dog fight? The cute one with the funny, white-tipped tail that belonged to Sandra Gonzales?"

It'd been only a few days back, so I remembered the case well. The teenage girl had rushed into the clinic with a three-month-old pooch bundled in a blood-smudged towel. Trying hard to control herself, she said, "I think Ranger was mauled by the dog next door. When I came home from school, he was just lying on the back porch, quiet and still like this."

We had cleaned and dressed the young pup's battle wounds, just as we've done so often for other dogs and cats. Even the softhearted Rachel left her reception desk, to come in and stroke the defenseless puppy's brow whenever he whimpered. Tracy administered the oral antibiotics, and Rachel carried the tiny pup to a soft bed in the kennel. In one way or another, each of us had handled or treated the little guy…and each of us had either saliva or blood from his tiny body on our hands and clothes.

"Is that the one, Rich? We were able to send him home the next day."

"You're right…well, Sandra's mom brought him back to us 'cause he was depressed and not eating. I stayed with him through the night, but then he suddenly became aggressive, trying to attack everything in his cage. He'd developed the final signs of the 'furious' form of rabies…and he died that morning, Doc. He didn't have much of a chance. I called Mrs. Gonzales first thing in the morning to let her know. She said her husband had killed a skunk a day after Ranger was first brought to us. It had been out during the day, wandering in haphazard circles by the tree stump where the puppy liked to play. So I asked her to bring the carcass in to us for testing. We needed to send both bodies on to Austin for analysis."

After another silence, he said, "…it turns out this wasn't a dog mauling after all…the 'lil pup must've had a run-in with the sick skunk. The report just came back…both tested *positive* for rabies. You know what we have to do now."

Taking a very slow, deep breath…I knew only too well what we had to do next. Any one of us could have contracted the virus through the tiniest nick in the skin, even a paper cut. Our entire staff and the Gonzales family had been exposed.

Oddly, Dr. Vest began laughing. "That'll mean twenty-one shots in the belly for everybody."

"Rich…how can you laugh?"

"…because I can't cry…we're scheduling the inoculations for everyone here. The Health Department requested we give the full series. But what are you goin' to do? You have no time to wait before starting the treatments."

We'd been worried something like this might happen. Several nearby communities had seen an increase in rabies. Rapid city growth had forced many species of wildlife from their burrows. Seeking safety in the only remaining areas, these animals are forced into smaller and smaller habitats. The sad results are overcrowding, disease, and starvation. Looking for food wherever they can find it, the misplaced creatures often search through rural barns and dwellings. Sandra and her family lived in such a farm community on the edge of town.

"I'll start my shots out here somewhere. I've got just one more colt to treat for Jake, then I'll figure somethin' out. But, Rich, I'm worried about Tracy, Rachel…and especially young Sandra. This is going to be rough on them. Make sure someone is with them during the procedures…okay?"

There were no physicians, drugstores, and certainly no vaccine doses for at least one hundred and fifty miles. But Hallie, always taking it upon herself to be everyone's savior, drove through the night to an Amarillo hospital where the medication was located. She also knew of a former childhood chum, now a retired doctor, who agreed to administer the shots to me.

Closing her café, Hallie picked me up at first light. It didn't seem to bother her that she'd had no sleep and would need to keep on driving that day, too. We took off to Dr. Vic Bronson's place…forty miles from Jake's ranch, where I'd been bunking during the corral work.

Hollering for us to come 'round back, Dr. Bronson held the screen door open as he invited me into his kitchen. Hallie decided to wait on the porch.

"You must be the fella needin' a shot. Ya want a sandwich first?" He was still in his bathrobe. And I noticed the doctor's hands tremble slightly as he reached for his glasses on the counter. Looking over his shoulder, I couldn't miss seeing his last medical license, thumbtacked to the pantry door. The date of issue was 1971. Victor was probably close to ninety years old. A little slumped, perhaps, but his voice was strong as he read from the package insert Hallie had given him. "Says here…to give this stuff in the belly…one shot daily in a clockwise pattern. Take off your shirt, boy." Then, handing me the needle, syringe, and vial, he added, "Here, son, you draw it up."

My nerves were frayed…and he closely watched me fumble with the thick medicine. Then, moving the peppershaker and the sugar bowl over to the sink, he motioned for me to lie on the table. The chilled Formica surface against my back made me shudder. Handing him the needle, I grasped his wrist to better focus his shaking aim. Looking at the needle…then at me, Dr. Bronson frowned and hesitated. "Dern it, son…this is gonna hurt." After gripping the table's edge and gritting my teeth, I told him to continue.

His hands ended up being sure and steady…but the pain was worse than I remembered. I just lay there for a few moments in semi-shock, trying to gather my wits. Then the good doctor helped me off the table, and I slowly made my way out the door, with Hallie at my side.

Turning to thank him, and to ask how much I'd owe for this…his answer was like everyone else's in these parts. "Well, son, I'll be needin' to see ya for the next few days. But when ya come back near Thanksgivin' for Hallie's big 84th birthday celebration, ya might see if you can find me a bumper for my Model-A there in the driveway." Closing the screen door, he added, "Ya *are* comin'… ain'tcha, son?"

Gingerly climbing into the truck, I called back, "You betcha, Doc…wouldn't miss it." Then, laying my head back, I was out like a light.

Knowing my recovery-nap would take a while…Hallie had thought to bring some of her famous homemade apple muffins to share with Doc Bronson. And the two old friends spent the rest of the morning laughing and gossiping over hot mugs of cinnamon coffee and the best muffins this side of the Rio Grande.

Like some sort of recurring dream, this scene was repeated day in and day out before I could even begin to think about heading back home to Dallas. What's worse, I never did get to taste Hallie's apple muffins.

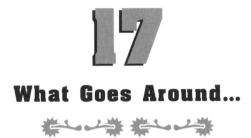

What Goes Around...

creeching sounds came from behind the barn. Thinking one of the animals was hurt...I ran toward the paddock. Oddly enough, it was only Dr. Vest... singing his heart out. Everyone for a block around got an earful of his off-key, plaintive rendition of tunes we couldn't even recognize. Making up his own words as he wailed away, we caught a snatch of "...ya gotta let your babies grow up to be cowboys, let 'em pick guitars and drive them ol' trucks, but don't make 'em be doctors 'n such..."

"Why is *he* so happy?" asked Tracy, covering her ears...as we watched him leading our old, dappled gray horse from the corral. Acting like he didn't have a care in the world, my partner continued to trash the lyrics of more well-known songs. Then he took to humming, clicking his heels together as though ready for a dance.

I didn't have the foggiest notion as to what put him in this mood. Wearing the same brown shirt he'd worn the day before, he moseyed toward us waving and smiling. His worn, wide-brimmed Stetson was snubbed all the way down to his ears. And we could see where the threads on the knees of his jeans had turned white from kneeling so often on the hard, rocky ground.

"Whoa...will ya take a look at that smile...he looks like he just swallowed a buzzard," exclaimed Tracy.

"Welp...at least he still looks sane," I chimed in.

Seemingly satisfied with himself, Rich wrapped the mare's lead rope around the hitching post at the back door. Then snapping his fingers to the tune in his head, he dusted sunflower pollen from his shirt and stepped inside.

"Okay...tell me, who spiked your coffee," Tracy asked.

"Nobody...can't a man have a good day?"

We both knew he had some sort of secret. But it was just like him to lead us on until we couldn't stand the suspense any longer.

"Where's our beautiful receptionist today," Rich asked, "...'cause I want to thank her for sending me to Jay Buchanan's this morning."

Now I knew something was seriously wrong. He either had malaria or was hallucinating from a sunstroke. I gulped hard. "*That attorney*...your ex-wife's divorce lawyer?"

Buchanan was known to be the most crooked gent around. "Rich, I can't believe this. *You* went to see Jay...after what he did to you? That sleazy character would sell scales to a fish before guttin' him alive."

My partner's smile broadened, and he could hardly contain himself. "What goes around…comes around. It's a go-ood day."

Following him through the large animal treatment area, while he grabbed a pair of hoof-nippers, I kept nagging, "C'mon …c'mon…what did you do?"

Walking out the back door, my partner said, "I'll tell ya, Doc…just as soon as I finish with Daisy here." Then, kneeling by the crippled mare's right foreleg, he snipped away a piece of chipped hoof from her foot. Daisy had suffered a tragic slab fracture, which left her knee unsound. Tending to her needs as if she was a Derby winner, Rich patted her neck and released the lead. "There, now, sweetheart…go eat some of that fresh grass," he murmured. Then he stopped to untangle a mat from her tail before Daisy limped off toward the pasture.

"Buchanan was playin' polo this mornin' when he called. About two weeks ago, he purchased a horse at a liquidation auction…you know—the *All Sales Final* kind. Anyway, he wanted to see me 'cause the gelding wasn't gaining any weight. I think ya know the horse he bought, Doc…it's Malibu Palm."

I knew the horse's medical history only too well. The Florida Thoroughbred was in worse physical condition than the retired Daisy, our lame mare. But, apparently, Jay didn't know he'd been swindled.

Rich then did his best imitation of Buchanan, mimicking the fellow's put-on Boston accent and nervous twitch: "I certainly know we've had our differences in the past, Richard, but will you come to the S&L Polo Club today and take a look at my new horse? I've been feeding him the very best alfalfa hay and oats, but…"

Dr. Vest had never been impressed with pretentiousness. And I couldn't help but imagine him arriving at the posh Polo Club and parking his dusty old truck right next to Jay's polished and buffed limousine. Picturing him in the club's lavish barn in his work-soiled clothes, I asked, "You actually went there to look at the grand old marshal, Malibu…whom I fondly call Jaws…'cause that former stud is as old as me and twice as ugly."

My partner went on to describe his encounter with Jay, saying that Buchanan complained his "…seven-year-old horse wasn't digesting his grain, his hair-coat was dull, his ribs were showing, and his hip bones protruded."

My surprise was that Malibu was still breathing, since I'd retired the old guy twelve years earlier.

Dr. Vest continued to relate his morning's conversation with Buchanan:

"When the gelding stretched his neck to the feed bin, I told Jay to watch very closely. Malibu munched a bite of the leafy green hay, then grinding his lower jawbone with a crushing action, and sucking…he spit out leafless stems.

'Did you get a pre-purchase exam on Malibu before buying the horse?' I calmly asked. After waiting for this so-called legal expert to answer, I asked again, 'Well, did ya?'

'What's that?' coughed Jay.

'It's an exam to test the soundness of wind and limb by a veterinarian like me…and necessary before you ever seal the deal.'"

Of course, the arrogant attorney wasn't going to believe Dr. Vest. "Look, I paid five thousand dollars for what they told me was the greatest polo horse around...and I insist you fix him."

To Buchanan's surprise, Rich simply put his hands in his back pockets, refusing to discuss it further. "Didn't you hear me?" the man snarled. My partner stood there quietly as Jay ranted on. "Money is no object, you know. Malibu is sluggish and even limps. I'm embarrassed by his appearance. Do I need to call another vet?"

At that moment, Rich could have taken Jay to the cleaners...just as Jay did to him a year earlier. Worming, vaccinations, blood chemistry profiles, cell counts, fecal exams, radiographs, hospitalization, repeated lameness tests, medications and vitamins, and more...could have all added up to a hefty bill. And Jay wouldn't have known the difference.

Shaking his head, Rich said, "I had him, Doc, right where I always wanted him...and it took everything in me not to drive the sonny-beech to the bank, and collect then and there. But ya know I can't profit on misery."

Instead, Rich told Jay to save his money. And after pointing to the stack of leafless alfalfa stems piled in the trough, he instructed, "Now, Mr. Buchanan, look there, and take a look right here in Malibu's mouth."

Jay obliged and saw the condition. "But that's unusual, isn't it?"

"Not for a thirty-four-year-old horse. The medical records are on file. Malibu has no molars...no teeth to eat with. He needs a special kind of soft diet 'cause he's a gummer."

I would have given anything to see the look on Jay's face when Rich gave him those facts. But Dr. Vest didn't tell us more. He just turned to go back inside, as Tracy and I followed behind. "Wait...so what happened then...and what about the horse?" we asked together.

"I told Jay that Malibu could live out his days in our back pasture in the company of other elders just like him. Buchanan didn't hesitate, but timidly agreed. And I walked away leaving him standing there...still bewildered."

My partner broke into song again, "...just don't let your babies grow up to be lawyers...and don't let 'em ever mess with the vet..."

Tracy couldn't stand it, "Stop...I'm sure glad ya never wasted your money on singin' lessons."

"When is Malibu joining us?" I asked.

"He'll be here tomorrow...the fourth horse to live happily ever after in our clinic's expanding Equine Senior Community. And the new pasture over at Meadow Creek can accommodate even more someday...don'tcha think?"

What could I say? There was never a time when I wasn't surprised and impressed with this man's rare character.

Columbo's Mystery

I t was bare and empty at the Meadow Creek facility in Flower Mound. Late one Friday afternoon, all five of the Twin Oaks pioneers—Dr. Vest, Rachel, Tracy, Billy and I—decided to check out the readiness of this new clinic. Only the most vital areas were complete: four ultra-modern examination suites, fully equipped and ready for action.

While Billy set about the task of assembling stainless steel cages in the wards, I decided to hang a Longhorn steer skull on the front wall of our reception area. For some reason, Rachel and Tracy took this moment to finally agree on something; they both expressed strong disgust at the thought I'd mess up the shiny new place.

"We need something rustic," I said, knowing all the while the skull didn't really belong in rooms exuding only the latest in modern technology. "It looks like a space station in here," I added, fondling the large, chipped relic that was once my Uncle Grump's prize bull.

I couldn't even get Billy's approval. Long ago given the title 'Head of Domestic Relations'—due to his prowess at diplomacy—Billy Chapman was smart enough to know who really ran our hospital.

Sirens suddenly shattered the quiet afternoon. "Whoa... that sounded close," my partner called from the other side of the room.

"Close?" said Rachel as she ran to the window, "They're right outside!"

A fireman in full protective gear—already covered with dripping soot—came bolting through our door.

"Danny, what are y'all doin' here...are we on fire?" yelled Rich. The large, stocky man behind the face shield was Dr. Vest's brother, whom I didn't immediately recognize.

In barely audible, broken breaths, Danny tried to speak, as he rushed over to Rich. "There was a...house fire. Here... quick...take him...here," and he extended the small bundle in his arms.

Before the exhausted fireman could fully catch his breath, Tracy had us ushered into an operating room—as Danny handed his brother a critically burned kitten he held wrapped in a wet towel.

The little body was lifeless—there was no pulse. "He's stopped breathing," I said, beginning cardiac massage. "Let's get some dopram, epinephrine and clippers here."

Struggling to put the cuffed tube down the baby kitten's windpipe, Dr. Vest said, "His larynx is swollen shut. By the length of his teeth, I'd guess 'im to be somewhere between ten months and a year old."

"His gums are blue, and his pupils are dilated and fixed," I noted as I parted the damp, matted hair on the cat's throat. My partner made a stab incision into the trachea to establish oxygen flow through the plastic canal. His hands moved away as I stooped to blow into the tube, dilating the lungs. "Airway's open," we said together.

Tracy pleaded, "C'mon, baby, breathe."

More shock-therapy medicines were needed, while rhythmic chest compression continued until I could thread a jugular catheter to administer respiratory and heart stimulants straight into the bloodstream.

"Is he alive?" asked Danny.

No one said anything. We paused for a second and felt for a heartbeat—there was none. After placing the flat face of my stethoscope on the kitten's thorax, and briefly jolting his rib cage, I thought I heard something. "It's faint...but it's beating...he's alive," I announced.

One breath was followed by two—then three. A twitch of his foot and movement of an eyelid made us feel better. But the cat was having a rough time. Coughing and gagging, his feeble groan turned into whimpers of pain. Visibly upset, Dr. Vest said, "If the flames didn't kill him, I reckon the pain from the burns could."

The little thing tried to struggle against his discomfort, but my partner cloaked the kitten's entire body in a swath of sterile cloth saturated with soothing ointment.

The concerned Danny had been hovering over our shoulders every minute. Rachel finally grabbed him by the arm to lead him out to his waiting truck, but he didn't want to leave. I'd always thought Dr. Vest and Danny were nothing alike. They didn't even resemble each other. But one thing was certain—they had the same kind of heart.

Adjusting the flow of supporting fluids, we slowly raised the towel to fully examine what had been done by the inferno —and winced. It was the first time we'd stopped long enough to see just how extensive his wounds were. The little guy looked like a partially fried, drowned rat. While life or death had been our primary worry, his future would be our next big concern.

"Whose cat is this, Danny?" Rich asked. "Danny...?"

Not answering, Danny stood there with his arms folded, as if in a trance. Patting his brother on the back, Dr. Vest asked again, "Danny...?"

Suddenly blurting, "What?" Danny didn't seem aware of Rich's question. His shoulders slumped from fatigue and his arms dropped to his sides, but his eyes were still riveted on the heart monitor's steady blips.

"...the only survivors were three cats," he finally said, "...we found the other two huddled under the back porch, but they were okay. My buddy took them to the adoption shelter on Grove Street."

Tracy's bluntness always cut right to the bone, "They're dead? His owners died in the fire? What happened?"

"I can't say much right now...it's all under investigation. But it appears to be a double homicide and arson." Then, tightening the strap on his helmet, he added, "It's best if I get back to my unit now. The guys are still out front waiting for me. Thanks, Docs." With a familiar nod to his brother, he shook my hand and pointed to the table where the small victim was lying. "Call me…let me know how he does, okay?"

As Danny left, Tracy took her customary, no-nonsense stance. Placing her hands on her hips, she asked, "So now what?…what are we gonna do with Charcoal here? In fact, that might be a good name for him."

"I kinda prefer 'Columbo'," said Rich, "…'cause of what Danny just said about the kitten being part of a real mystery they'd be tryin' to investigate." Instinctively, we felt the cat's new name was perfect. What we didn't know, then, was just how involved the little feline would ultimately become in the unfolding developments of this strange case.

Seventy percent of Columbo's black and white forequarters had suffered third-degree burns, and nothing but patches of seared skin covered the raw muscles over his rump and down his back legs. One ear and two toes were missing. And he had no whiskers. Our major cause for concern was the corneal scarring caused by the intense heat from the flames. The cat would always be partially blind. Visibly shaken, Dr. Vest closed his eyes—sighing. I knew what he was thinking. We both knew it would take months for the kitten to mend. We also knew what Tracy had been thinking—would it have been kinder to put him to sleep?

At times like this, each of us felt the same: If a wounded animal could be kept comfortable, we'd continue to do our best to help it survive.

"If he makes it," I said, "…the kitten can become Meadow Creek's mascot. By the time it opens, he should be healed. But first things first. Billy, can you please make a special bed for Columbo, and put it next to the desk in my office?"

Before we headed home to Twin Oaks, I grabbed the Longhorn skull, figuring I'd hang it there instead of the new place. It would fit in better at the old reception room, anyway. Tracy and Rachel never said another word about it.

Columbo's bandages were changed twice daily—and he showed good, steady progress. When our neighbors heard about the disfigured cat, we were inundated with dozens of offers to adopt him. These caring folks knew the little guy would never be beautiful, which made their response all the more heart-warming. But it had been already decided... we wanted him to be with us.

As Columbo became bigger and stronger, his sweet personality took shape. Developing a very gregarious nature, he'd amble through our offices visiting everyone who came in—even the dogs. No one knew why, but he especially took to the large retrievers—particularly one. Whenever Jesse, a mature golden, came through the door, Columbo knew it and would come barreling out from wherever he was to rub his head in Jesse's neck, mewing and purring at the same time. Jesse seemed to feel the same way, and the two would romp and tumble around in the middle of the reception area—providing entertainment for our waiting clients.

The endearing cat's preferred lookout spot for meeting and greeting clients was on the counter of Rachel's reception desk. He'd take his naps there, too, on one of the few things Rachel ever tried to sew...a quilted pillow-bed. She even managed to create a green-patterned design of letters, with COLUMBO sewn in—a little crooked—but personal all the same.

People loved the little mystery cat with so much character. He graced our clinic for years, remaining as much a part of our daily lives and our ups and downs as any indispensable member of our close family.

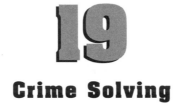

Crime Solving

Sheets of summer lightning greeted our descent into Dallas. As we began dropping through turbulent black clouds...my imagination got the best of me. Nervously clenching the armrests, I was ready for anything. This wasn't going to be an easy landing.

"At last, there are the runway lights!" a lady's voice rang out. The clasp of the seatbelt dug into my waist when the engines roared into reverse. With all the bumping and tossing about, I couldn't tell if we'd landed or not until the unmistakable smell of seared rubber filled the cabin. I silently thanked the pilot for safely getting us back on the ground.

Taxiing up to Gate 24, we expected to see the flexible tentacle of the jet-way attach itself to our departure door...but only empty runway appeared. The Captain's voice interrupted our restlessness to quickly leave the planes' confines. "Welcome to Dallas and Fort Worth. It's 12:05 A.M., Central Standard time. And the temperature is 99 degrees. We apologize for the delays due to rain, and look forward to your flying with us again. We may need to wait here a little while longer until they're ready for us. Thanks again for your patience, folks."

With dozens of planes landing and jockeying for position, it became apparent the wait would be more than a 'little while'. Laying my head back and closing my eyes, my thoughts drifted. It had been only a few weeks since the fire, and I wondered how our little burn victim, Columbo, was making out in my absence.

Then suddenly it came to me—I'd seen our new mascot before. Something about the weather and the sounds all jogged my memory. A few months ago, on a night like this—rainy and hot—I'd treated him for an abscess on the side of his neck. I couldn't remember the owner's name—but I'd been struck by her unusually long, straight black hair. Dark-skinned and pretty, I wondered where she was from, and asked about her slight accent. Other than saying she was born in South America, she didn't mention a region or any other details. She kept calling the kitten Deeno, and I thought it might be a Spanish term. The woman didn't offer much in the way of conversation. But I was sure Rachel would have more information in her old appointment book.

Arriving home at 3:00 A.M., still hyper from the rough flight home, there was no way I'd be able to sleep. Tossing and turning, I decided to just get up and go straight to the clinic. By getting in at dawn, I'd beat the rest of the crew to work. But every light was blazing when I got there. And Tracy was swearing at someone in the kennels, "Dammit, Adam! Somebody catch that fur-ball."

"I've got 'im," Dr. Vest hollered. "Yowch!...now he's loose again."

This wasn't exactly the quiet morning I expected. I'd almost forgotten we'd agreed to neuter and spay A.J. Hall's two half-wild, adopted cats—Adam and Eve. Our most cantankerous client had a way of claiming he needed his appointments first thing in the morning.

My partner yelled again, as Adam bit his arm and then jumped on top of one of the kennel cages. I could already hear A.J. saying. "Oh, what's wrong with you?...they're friendly." The tattered green-plaid shirt the horse trader always wore would be covered with mustard stains from a week ago, and the stumpy cigar he kept unlit in the corner of his mouth only added to his know-it-all attitude. This ornery character managed to rile me more than any other client we've ever had.

But I'd forget about A.J. right now, and pitch in with the dilemma at hand. Adam was loose in the clinic. And his littermate, Eve, was nervously pacing in her cage. We needed to take care of them both before other clients began arriving.

Trying to find a way out, the year-old kitten raced through the clinic, knocking over bottles of medicine and managing to send a microscope catapulting on its side. When the black and white feline came streaking down the hallway, I attempted to block his escape. Instead, after leaving claw marks across the toes of my good, black dress boots, he leapt over to the front counter, sending medical records flying in every direction. Rachel screamed...and Adam sprang into the air over the benches, only to turn, run back down the hall and dart into the large animal surgical suite. Now we had him. We quickly closed huge steel doors behind him. The little eight-pound tomcat would have trouble destroying anything in this special room. Even a thousand-pound colt couldn't put a dent into it.

"Well, he's trapped now," Dr. Vest laughed, "...but I'd rather wrestle a badger than an angry cat. Maybe we should call Fred Landsberry to work his soothing magic on him."

"Adam's just young and scared," I said, "...he'll come around."

Realizing he was trapped, the ransacking kitten squalled at the top of his lungs. Then, after a few moments, he quieted in the partial darkness of the room.

"See?" I exclaimed, "He's okay now."

I must admit, at times like these, I was glad we'd spared no expense in planning this large-animal surgical suite. It was built to withstand anything from wild beasts to explosions. In case of a tornado, I'd head there first. The eight-inch cement block walls were braced with rebar, and layered with thick vinyl coverings. Even the three-ton hydraulic surgery table could be recessed flush with the padded flooring. The engineers had thought of just about everything. But as we discovered, small flying animals weren't anticipated. From the viewing window, we watched Adam jump onto the large surgical lamps suspended from the solid steel rafters and start to swing back and forth on the five-ton hoist used to maneuver anesthetized horses into position.

The little guy ended up falling from the twelve-foot-high ceiling rafters. Shaken, but not hurt, Adam began sniffing around and exploring the immense room.

Realizing it would take some time for the kitten to calm down, I went out to our barn to check on a few of the mares. While changing a leg dressing on a paint filly, Tracy and Rachel's loud laughter echoed out from the clinic. They were peering through the window at Dr. Vest, who'd decided to take matters into his own hands.

I did a double take, not believing the lengths my partner would go to in order to get a job done. He stood in the middle of the octagonal surgical suite dressed in what looked like gladiator attire. Spinning around and around trying to catch Adam, he was encumbered by the restrictions of his weighty garb—which happened to be the padded chest protector of my son's Little League catcher's outfit. Shin guards covered the fronts of his legs and, of course, his face was hidden by the steel cage of the catcher's mask.

I couldn't resist needling the warrior, "Need any help in there, Spartacus?"

Billy got into the act by yelling over my shoulder, "Catch 'im in your glove, Dr. V."

After a few swift moves, Dr. Vest pinned Adam to the mat and hollered for some sedation. Dashing in, I gave the injection into the cat's leg muscle. Rich released his grip, and Adam ran just a few steps before crouching and dropping to his side—sound asleep, and finally ready for surgery.

Dr. Vest, always the showman, placed the tiny cat in the middle of the giant hydraulic table. And it was evident he planned on performing the neutering right there instead of in our surgery room for small animals. Gears turned, the platform rose...and bright beams illuminated the area. "Doc, I'll 'fix' Adam in here if you'll spay Eve in the next room. Then we'll get 'em both done at the same time."

Tracy wrapped Eve in a towel while I administered the dose of anesthesia. Preparing for the surgery, I muttered, "Who else but A.J. would name his scrapping cats Adam and Eve?"

My partner yelled from the other room, "Well, that ol' coot must have a soft spot…'cause he adopted those kittens right after the fire at the Milligan's place."

"You're kidding…where your brother found Columbo?" In amazement, I looked down at Eve. "Well, I'll be dang…." She had the same black mustache marking as both Adam and Columbo…although Columbo's was scarred. The kittens were all about the same age. And both Adam and Eve were adopted from the Grove Street kennel where Danny told us he'd taken the survivors of the fire.

It seemed impossible, but it all came together. The three cats were kin—no doubt about it.

I focused on completing the surgery for Eve, but my thoughts were racing. I would check old files with Rachel to be certain…but I remembered. The lady's name was Lynnette, Lynnette Romero. And she called the mother cat Windy. Tying off one of the last surgical knots on Eve, I yelled out, "Adam and Eve's mother must've died in the fire… but Danny didn't say anything about finding four cats."

Thinking we might have an answer to the cause of the Milligan fire, I said, "Tracy…listen…we can help Danny with that homicide investigation…and maybe even tell him where the Romero woman can be found."

In the process of cleaning Eve's closed incision, Tracy looked over at me as though I were nuts. "What are you talking about, Doc?" At that, Dr. Vest and Rachel appeared in the doorway.

Removing my latex gloves, I announced to the crew, "The picture is clear to me. There was Dustin, the younger of the two Milligan brothers—and Roy, who was my age. But Roy moved away years ago. Dustin married a young Cajun girl from New Orleans. She had no family ties, so they lived with his grandmother in the family's white, two-story frame house. I should have recognized the clues."

Carried away by my own cleverness, I asked Rachel to get Danny on the phone for me. "No, I won't," she said, "…'cause I think you're crazy!"

Dialing Danny at the fire department myself, I blurted out, "Danny, didn't you say two people died in that fire last month?"

"Yeah, Doc…I did…but why do you ask?"

Sounding a bit melodramatic, I then asked, "Was it a male and a female?"

"It was…but the investigation is still going on. In fact, I was talking to Sheriff Simon about it this morning."

"It was Roy and his grandma," I declared.

After an awkward silence, I realized Danny wasn't supposed to be discussing police business with anyone. But he had to find out what I knew. "Wait, Doc…don't tell me anything more," he said. "I'll meetcha at Twin Oaks in an hour."

Danny, Sheriff Dave Simon, and a detective I'd never met showed up in an unmarked car an hour later. They parked at our back entrance, and I ushered them into my office. But I wondered why they were putting on such a show of secrecy. I'd known Dave for years, and he'd been out to the clinic often. Just elected to his third term, 'Sheriff Dave', as the kids called him, epitomized the B-movie concept of the good ol' boy town sheriff. His uniform was too tight, and his pudgy beer-gut hung out over the top of his trousers. Slow talking and slow moving, I'd always thought his unruffled attitude made him perfect for the job. The general gossip around town contended that the large, old-style firearm tied to his belt was just for show. And we were all sure he never fired it. Still, knowing him to be patient and thorough...I was glad Danny had brought him by.

Detective Jerry Standish had a very dismissive attitude toward me, acting as though this visit was a waste of his time, especially when I began spouting off about a mama cat called Windy and her three kittens. Danny gave me a supportive nod when I relayed what happened after the fire. And he told us one other cat was found at the scene, but had succumbed to smoke inhalation.

I continued on to explain the happenings of the previous year. "When I asked Lynette to come back in five days with Deeno, who is now Columbo, she said, ' I'm not sure I can, I'm awfully busy.' She never returned."

"But just before I left for Chicago last week, I ran into Dustin Milligan at the hardware store and asked how his grandmother was doing. I joked with him, saying his wonderful grandma must be a hundred years old by now. And Dustin just mumbled, '...she almost made it, too.' At the time, I didn't know what to make of his comment. I mentioned to him I'd seen his brother Roy recently, and he was looking good. Dustin didn't say anything. But he kept fidgeting with his shirt buttons, then made an excuse to leave for some appointment."

I tried to recall my brief visit with Roy, which was a few weeks before the fire, and remembered something he had said.

"He told me he was back in town temporarily to help out the family, since Dustin and Lynette's rock-cutting business was in some sort of financial trouble."

Sliding to the edge of his chair, Sheriff Simon interrupted, "Lynnette Romero is also Lynn Landers, Linda McQueen, and Lucy Bell. They are all aliases. Her real name is Natalie Corwin."

Suddenly, what I'd been telling them didn't seem so foolish. Jerry Standish, now warming up to me, continued with the information they had so far. "Natalie was an orphan, who ended up being raised by one of the captains of a Mississippi steamboat. He was found drowned about a year back...and the case is still open."

The sheriff decided to let us in on the rest. "This Natalie is a tough one...she and Dustin were dealing cocaine and heroine for years. Dustin's brother must have found out about it..."

"And they killed Roy and his grandma?" Danny asked.

"So, they *were* murdered?" I repeated.

Nodding his head toward both of us, Dave said, "I'm afraid so. The fire was set to hide the facts."

This confirmation saddened me. Roy and his grandmother were good people. And I hated hearing that Dustin had taken such a gruesome turn. After hesitating a moment, I was almost afraid to say more. "It's possible I have some clues y'all might need to find 'em."

This time Dave Simon and Detective Standish didn't think I was stupid when I offered my theory. "I went back through our records. In her thoroughness, Rachel had asked for and jotted down the names of Deeno's littermates. They were called Frisco and Charles. And we already know the mother cat was Windy.

In other words, these could be names for Big D or Dallas, San Francisco, Chicago and Charleston. Do you think that's too far-fetched? Could they have contacts there?"

The detective jumped to his feet, and Dave leaned over to shake my hand, saying, "Thanks, Doc…this isn't as wild as you may think…and could narrow our search."

We didn't hear from anyone for a few weeks. In the meantime, Adam and Eve had gone home with A.J. But he'd never know that the appearance of his two cats at the clinic sparked my memory, and may have led to the solving of a murder mystery.

On a Tuesday, at the close of the day, I answered a call on my way out the door. It was Danny with some news. All he said was, "Tell Columbo, our mystery cat…thanks for all the clues."

"You're kidding, right? You mean my theories were actually true? You've got to be kidding."

Danny laughed, "Nope, I'm not kidding. They got 'em and Sheriff Simon is bringing 'em back to Texas for trial. They apprehended Dustin at Pier 39 in San Francisco, and arrested Natalie at the Ritz Hotel an hour later. They were registered under the names Lindsay and Dusty Braddock. And they had enough drugs on 'em to sink a ship. Good work, Doc, the case is solved."

Maybe someday I'll tell ol' A.J. Hall that our sweet mascot and his two ruffian-cats are related…then again, maybe I won't.

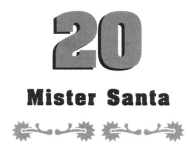

Mister Santa

winkling blue and green mini-lights adorned an artificial tree in the pharmacy, helping to brighten our spirits…despite the unseasonal 85-degree heat. Enjoying the pretense that this was a traditional winter's Christmas Eve, Rachel and Tracy giddily exchanged gifts of perfume, while I handed out holiday bonus checks to Dr. Vest, Billy, and the girls.

With everyone feeling festive, and ready to bolt out of the door at five o'clock…Dr. Vest asked us to wait. One more patient was due in—his next door neighbor, Jackie Flynn. She was out looking for a puppy to give her kids for Christmas, and would be coming to the clinic for its first checkup.

At the sound of the chiming doorbell, Rachel hustled to the front desk. And we overheard her cooing, "Oh…isn't he the cutest thing."

After extending Christmas greetings to Jackie, we all took turns cuddling the tiny white and tan puppy. As I held up the five-week-old Jack Russell Terrier to admire his unusual markings, especially the heart-shaped brown circle around just one eye, Jackie proudly said, "His name is Mister Santa."

The endearing bundle of energy ran across the floor to Tracy, his ears flapping…and his stubby legs working so fast that his long body wobbled. "He rocks like a seesaw," she said, "…the tan patch on his back looks like a 'lil saddle."

Mister Santa coughed, a dry hack, then began tugging on Dr. Vest's pant leg. "Brave little devil, ain'tcha," Tracy said, scooping the playful runt up into her arms. "I could just squeeze the puddin' out of you." His tail was wagging a mile a minute, and his long pink tongue smacked Tracy on the kisser. "Why you're just a love-crazy wiggle-worm." Smothering the precious little guy against her neck with a hug, she laughed when the pup nipped at one of her dangling snowman earrings.

Looking over at me, Jackie said, "I saw him in the window of the pet store, and just couldn't pass him up. But, Doc…I need to be sure he's healthy before my kids see Mister Santa tomorrow mornin'."

I told her that Dr. Vest would be doing the exam, "But it does sound like he might have a touch of kennel cough."

With straight-cut blond hair pushed back behind her ears, the young woman had an all-American-girl look. And though the single mother of three had a good job as a secretary for a local construction company, it was hard for her to make ends meet. Her company had held its office party that noon, and Jackie was still wearing a nametag-ornament pinned to her white wool turtleneck sweater. Apparently she, too, was trying to get into the spirit of a snowy Christmas that didn't exist in Texas.

My partner chased the shorthaired pup from one end of the exam table to the other until he could hold him long enough to listen to his heart and lungs. There was no congestion, and his temperature was normal. But a choking hack would come on after the slightest surge of play or tracheal compression.

"Is that kennel cough serious?" asked his new owner.

Prying the dog's jaws open to check his throat, my partner explained, "It's a type of highly infectious bronchitis. And at this time of year, we see tons of it…especially in pets coming from shelters, pet stores, or boarding kennels. It seldom makes 'em very sick, but they'll cough up phlegm for a while, as if they have a sore throat."

"I've seen a half-dozen cases today," I added. "Still, it shouldn't be ignored."

Agreeing, Rich said, "Pneumonia can develop when their resistance is down…so we'll put Mister Santa on a cough sedative and some oral antibiotics."

Knowing Jackie had spent her Christmas savings on her youngsters, he took extra time to discuss the treatment options. On the most exciting day of the year, the puppy was going to a strange new household with three young children. He was going to be played with, carried and chased to the point of exhaustion. Realizing this would create added stress, Dr. Vest and Jackie agreed to help bolster the pup's recovery and stamina with an injection of penicillin and vitamins.

Every muscle in Mister Santa's body wiggled with glee when Tracy clutched him to her chest. Again, the joyful pup tried to chew off her earring. While I offered him a dog biscuit as a distraction, Dr. Vest popped a minimal dose into his hindquarter without the pup noticing.

"He thought you were playing," said Jackie, as she gathered the squirming ball of fur in her hands and kissed him, branding him on the cheek with a smudge of pink lipstick. "Here," said Rachel, who couldn't resist using a bit of her new perfume, "... we'll make him smell pretty." Mister Santa ducked away from the fragrant mist by cuddling deep under Jackie's cradled arm. With his head tucked under her sweater, he thought he was hiding but his rump wagged his tail like it was a signal flag. It was 5:25...and Rachel tallied the bill while Dr. Vest began counting out the prescription pills for Jackie to administer to Mister Santa during the next week.

Then...a scream shattered the air. "DOCS!"

My partner dropped the pill vial and ran to the front desk. Something awful had just taken place, and I rushed forward to see Dr. Vest snatching Mister Santa from Jackie's outstretched arms.

"What happened, Rachel?"

In shock, her words spilled over one another. "I don't know...I don't know. He was fine...then suddenly his eyes rolled back and he collapsed."

Jackie's face froze, "...he just went limp."

Quickly using his stethoscope, Rich couldn't find a heartbeat. I looked at the pup's pale gums and opened his eyelids, but there was no sign of life...only a dead stare. As I began cardiac massage, my partner tried mouth-to-mouth lung dilation...and we watched for a breath—to no avail. We kept trying. Tracy reached for the crash cart, and my partner administered respiratory and cardiac stimulants sublingually at first, then straight into the jugular vein—but nothing. "C'mon, son," Rich pleaded …but words didn't help either.

Mister Santa was dead—from an allergic reaction to penicillin. There was no other explanation. I'd seen it happen only once before—in a horse. The odds were extreme, but there have been rare cases where it was known to have occurred.

In disbelief, Dr. Vest kept staring down at the table, patting the limp little body as if he could awaken it.

Everyone, including Billy, stood in the doorway…stunned and quiet.

Jackie, sensing that Rich felt responsible, broke the silence. "Dr. Vest, it wasn't your fault. There was no way you could know."

She was right. But I knew how my partner felt. Three years earlier, I'd given penicillin to a three-week-old colt, and he hit the deck. I wanted to bang my head against a concrete wall…every cell in my body hurt.

We'd given an untold number of penicillin injections over the years. But for us, even these two adverse reactions were too many. Motioning for Rich and Tracy to follow me into my office, I quickly tore a blank check from my bankbook, and handed it to Tracy. "Here…take Jackie back to the pet store before it closes."

We heard Jackie declining, but Tracy was firm. "Now…you'd better come with me. You don't know these doctors like I do. They might figure out some way to bring a huge St. Bernard down your chimney…whether you have a fireplace or not."

As the door closed behind them, Dr. Vest yelled, "We'll be right here waiting for ya."

Asking my disheartened partner to follow me into the kennels, I pointed toward all the dogs. We were filled to capacity for the holiday weekend. Over a hundred 'boarding pets' of every shape, size and color were barking at the top of their lungs. I was blunt. "Tomorrow morning at 6 o'clock, you, me and Billy will swear we'd rather be somewhere else...especially on Christmas. But we'll be here, putting their needs before our own. All we can do is our best. And if you lose one, you've got to get up and save two."

My short speech was overly dramatic, but he got the point.

Twenty minutes later, Tracy hollered, "We're back!"

Standing in the exam room, Tracy and Jackie were each holding a puppy. "Two...two?...me and my big mouth," I laughed.

"They gave us two for the price of one," Tracy happily explained. "They were the last two puppies in the shop...and one is a littermate to Mister Santa. See? He has the same markings. And we couldn't leave this other pup all by himself over Christmas," whined our technician, as she snuggled with the long-haired, black fuzzy mutt.

Giving me a knowing look, my partner shook his head, "...like ya said, for every one down, save two."

Both puppies were hacking with the same kennel cough. While Rich examined the Jack Russell, I listened to the other's chest. "Hey, Jackie"...noted Dr. Vest, "this is a female."

Chiming in, I added, "...and this one's a male."

"I know," said Jackie, "I'm calling her Angel and him..."

Administering a shot of penicillin to each pup, Rich again walked in to the pharmacy to count out two vials of antibiotic pills. When he returned, Jackie completed her sentence, "…and I'm calling the boy 'Doc'."

"After me?" I asked.

"No," she sweetly corrected, "…after my good friend 'n neighbor, Dr. Vest."

Between barking and coughing, Angel and Doc cavorted and played with one another under our watchful eyes. Fortunately, neither showed any reaction to the medication.

Smiling with relief, my partner stroked the mongrel terrier and looked at us. "Merry Christmas eve…and Doc, Billy, I'll see you two in the mornin'."

It was now seven o'clock. Hesitating at the door on his way out, Rich asked, "Jackie, how are you goin' to keep the kids from seeing the puppies tonight?"

Tracy boldly answered for Jackie, "…'cause they'll be stayin' at *your* house. It's a perfect plan. You're right next door."

My amiable partner obliged without saying another word, and—holding a pup under each arm—carried the two wiggling Christmas gifts out into the warm night air, setting them side by side on the blanketed front seat of his truck.

Jackie looked worried. "Those pups will be playin' all night long…do ya think Dr. Vest will get any sleep?"

"Nope…but somehow, I don't think he'll mind," I said, shooing everyone out the door. But Jackie poked her head back inside, and I read her lips as she softly whispered *thank you… thank you.*

"Ho…ho…ho," I sang out…"Merry Christmas to y'all."

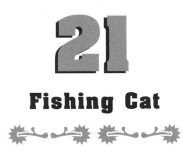

Fishing Cat

edical records cluttered Rachel's desk. With mussed hair, and her blue clinic smock splattered with soapy water...she was definitely not herself. Dr. Vest barely looked up, exiting one exam room to quickly enter another. The fatigue was showing on my partner's drawn face.

It was well after 6:00 P.M., and I hadn't expected to see anyone but staff at Twin Oaks. The reception area was still crowded with two springer spaniels, a black Lab, and an impatient Siamese cat. When not hiding under the blanket on her owner's lap, the irritable cat spent her time angrily hissing at the Lab, who just wouldn't leave her alone.

I'd just had a full, harrowing day at the Meadow Creek clinic and then out at Pete Samuel's ranch. So I didn't come in to work, but to talk about upcoming interviews for needed staff. The five of us were now trying to operate two clinics at once.

But the chaos here and backed-up appointments would probably continue if someone didn't jump in to help.

"Dr. Vest is with Peanut and Tim Bollen in Room Two," Rachel said, "...and I don't know why 'cause Peanut's stitches were just removed this mornin', but Tim did say somethin' about a string..." Before she could finish, I walked in to see for myself. My partner showed obvious relief when I assured him I'd stay until all the waiting critters had gone home.

Tim Bollen appeared embarrassed. "I didn't plan on seein' y'all again quite so soon." His friendly little shorthair cat contentedly lay on her side purring when Dr. Vest began his examination. Having spayed her recently, he began running his fingers across the soft, clipped fur of her belly, when Tim interrupted, "Oh, it's not her stomach...not exactly...," Tim said hoarsely, about to lose his voice. "Sorry, Docs...but I think I caught a cold on the lake."

Puzzled, my partner and I looked at one another, thinking the same thing. *Why did Tim bring Peanut back in today?* The incision site was healed, and her hair was growing back. Just then, Peanut took a playful swipe with her paw at a fine strand of nylon twine on the table. But there was no twine on the table. It had come from the corner of her mouth. "Wait a minute...Tim, is that what I think it is?" asked Dr. Vest. "What did she swallow?"

Stammering, Tim tried to explain. "I'd just come home from fishin' and was unloading my gear, when Peanut ran into the garage and gulped the baited hook on my rod before I could stop her." Nervously running his thumbs up and down his red suspenders, he grimaced. "I can't believe she ate the whole thing."

At that, he leaned over and scratched the oranged-striped feline behind her ears.

When I took her face in my hands, Peanuts stared at me with her bright green eyes…then extended her front paws to push me away. Since we knew the radiant piece of curved, barbed brass would be easy to locate, Dr. Vest carried the unsuspecting cat into the X-ray room. A two-dimensional radiograph could produce several images, including black for air, gray for water and organs, and white for bones *and* metal. Thinking this was all play, Peanut became overly frisky, darting off in every direction as Rich kept bringing her back, trying to adjust her body in different positions on the table in order to take the pictures.

"You'll obviously be here awhile," I laughed, "…so I'll go check in on Gus. Rachel says he might need a blood sample drawn. " Entering the next exam room, Mellie Daniels immediately voiced her concern.

"Doc, Gus isn't very dandy…he's got a really dry cough, and Dr. Vest told me I should bring him in."

Setting the four-year-old collie's file on the counter, I bent down to schmooze with him, while stroking his well-groomed tan and white coat. "Are you a good boy, Gus?" Straining, I lifted the eighty-pound male onto the table as he twisted uncomfortably. "Are ya?" His back legs were splayed behind him and his forepaws gripped the table's edge. Though he knew and trusted me, Gus was still panting with nervousness. Adjusting the rubber earpieces of the stethoscope, I listened intently…hearing a muffled cardiac murmur and unsettling sounds deep in the tissues of his lungs.

"Mellie, has Gus ever been tested for heartworms or been given tablets for heartworm prevention?"

The distinguished elderly woman was unusually frank. "He was tested as a puppy, but I quit givin' him the pills. I know heartworm is carried by mosquitoes…but Gus is an inside dog."

I'd always found it easy talking with Mellie. And though reserved, she was intelligent and direct. So I was honest with her. "Unless Gus knows how to flush the toilet by himself, he's not an inside dog. And his long hair doesn't guarantee protection, either." After drawing a small blood sample from the vein in Gus's forearm, I told the charming lady we'd know more as soon as I examined it under the microscope.

Unfortunately, it was immediately apparent—this was a parasite of the cardiovascular system. A mosquito can pick up the immature parasite during a blood meal from an infected dog, after which the parasite develops into larvae within two weeks. When the mosquito bites another dog, the larvae are deposited. They mature in two to three months, becoming thread-like adult worms that damage the heart and pulmonary artery. Within four to six months, even more are produced. As a result, the animal slowly dies as a result of congestive heart failure. This happened much too often. And I sometimes felt like posting banners all over the city, announcing the facts and urging owners to get the easy preventive treatments.

Mellie had already guessed what I would say. "He's got heartworms, doesn't he? He's not going to die…is he, Doc?"

"The disease is treatable, Mellie. But without therapy, the worms will drill holes in Gus's heart muscle and the pump will quit working."

This quiet, obedient dog was the woman's only companion. Her husband had died in an auto accident just a year earlier. In a breaking voice, she quietly asked if we could please start treatment right away. "Leave Gus with us, and Dr. Vest will begin the injections tomorrow…because I'll be over at our new clinic."

Hugging Gus tightly, and planting a kiss on his forehead…Mellie walked out front with Rachel. I took the collie into the kennels, but not before calming him down by giving him a few treats to munch on.

* * * * *

Emerging from the darkroom with Peanut's radiographs still dripping, my partner held them up for all to see. "Thar' she blows!" The bright metal gleamed through like a silver dollar.

With Tracy now over at Meadow Creek, Rachel was doing double duty until new staff arrived. And Dr. Vest enjoyed heckling her. "Put a bow in your Texas big-hair, Rachel…'cause we're goin' fishin'."

Surgery wasn't scheduled this late in the evening, but the hook had to come out right away. Tim Bollen nodded his consent and Dr. Vest proceeded.

During Peanut's surgery, I took on our waiting clients, medicating the Siamese for a slight respiratory ailment and vaccinating the spaniels and the Lab. The treatments for these last few patients didn't take long, and my partner was still in surgery when I waved goodbye to the still-hissing Siamese. This visit had been too traumatic for the gorgeous cat. I gave her owner one of our small carriers, hoping she'd use it in the future since it would give her sensitive pet the privacy it needed.

Locking the front door, I joined my partner in the surgical suite. He was smiling. "Ya know, we're lucky...the sharp tips of that sickle-shaped lure hadn't yet perforated the wall of Peanut's stomach."

Rachel was giggling, holding a small cup of water in her hand. "Look...this is weird...the fish is still alive." She spoke too soon, and the minnow drew his last breath as Dr. Vest asked for my assistance in stitching Peanut's abdominal muscles closed.

Swirling the fish-cup, Rachel added, "Docs, any sooner and you could've saved two lives for the price of one." I'd spent so much time at Meadow Creek lately, I'd forgotten how much I missed her attempts at humor.

At the end of Peanut's fishing expedition, Dr. Vest carried the cute one-year-old with the huge green eyes to her recovery cage. Then, turning to me, he began hinting again. "Ya know, Doc...that minnow would look best mounted next to the bladder-stone paperweight on my desk...*if* my office was also at Meadow Creek."

"I know we originally planned for you to stay here...but plans change. That's why I came back here tonight," I said. "Finish treating Gus, and as soon as both he and Peanuts go home, pack your bags and join me at the new place. And Rachel, get your files in order...'cause you're comin' with us, too. We'll hire a new staff for Twin Oaks from the group of interns coming in next week."

At that moment, a key turned and the front door of Twin Oaks flew open followed by a strong gust of wind...and Tracy.

She's the only one who knew I wanted to keep the team together. Giving her a signal that I'd just announced the happy decision, she jokingly hollered like a staff sergeant, "Okay, let's pack up and move out...move-it...move-it...onward to Meadow Creek. We've got people to see, places to be, and animals to treat."

I thought to myself, "Dang...why didn't I say that?"